Identity in the COVID-19 Years

Identity in the COVID-19 Years

Communication, Crisis and Ethics

Rob Cover

BLOOMSBURY ACADEMIC
NEW YORK • LONDON • OXFORD • NEW DELHI • SYDNEY

BLOOMSBURY ACADEMIC
Bloomsbury Publishing Inc
1385 Broadway, New York, NY 10018, USA
50 Bedford Square, London, WC1B 3DP, UK
29 Earlsfort Terrace, Dublin 2, Ireland

BLOOMSBURY, BLOOMSBURY ACADEMIC and the Diana logo
are trademarks of Bloomsbury Publishing Plc

First published in the United States of America 2024

For legal purposes the Acknowledgements on p. viii constitute an extension
of this copyright page.

Cover design: Eleanor Rose
Cover illustration by Annabel Hewitson

Bloomsbury Publishing Inc does not have any control over, or responsibility for,
any third-party websites referred to or in this book. All internet addresses given
in this book were correct at the time of going to press. The author and publisher
regret any inconvenience caused if addresses have changed or sites have ceased
to exist, but can accept no responsibility for any such changes.

A catalog record for this book is available from the Library of Congress.

ISBN:	HB:	978-1-5013-9367-9
	PB:	978-1-5013-9368-6
	ePDF:	978-1-5013-9370-9
	eBook:	978-1-5013-9369-3

Typeset by Integra Software Services Pvt. Ltd.

To find out more about our authors and books visit www.bloomsbury.com
and sign up for our newsletters.

For Jeff Williams, who in interdependency and entanglement shares the COVID years with me.

Contents

Acknowledgements

Struggling to understand the implications for identity and belonging of a new virus and the disruptions to everyday sociality cannot, of course, occur in isolation, despite the long periods of social distancing since the beginning of the COVID-19 pandemic. I owe a significant debt of gratitude to many people with whom I talked about this topic over several years, including Vera and Ian Cover, Barb and Roger Williams, Peter Aggleton, Ros Prosser and Veronika Petroff, Chris Beasley, Lisa Waller, Lukas Parker, Duc Dau, Ashleigh Haw, Charlotte Young, Katia Ostapets, Sharon Greenfield and dozens of strangers in an array of settings.

I acknowledge the support of the Humanities Research Centre at the Australian National University, where a funded visiting fellowship afforded the time, facilities and scholarly engagement to think through many aspects of COVID-19, identity and belonging – particular thanks to Kylie Message-Jones and Ibrahim Abraham.

This book was written on the unceded lands of the Wurundjeri, Taungurung and Ngunnawal peoples, the traditional owners, the elders – past, present and emerging – to whom I pay my respects.

Introduction: Stories of rupture and resilience in a pandemic

Introduction

A week before the city I was living in went into lockdown as the key strategy to prevent the early spread of the little-understood SARS-CoV-2, my university issued a strict work-from-home policy, with twenty-four hours' notice to collect any items we might need for several weeks from our offices. I saw the email at about 11 pm, and realizing that I might need several trips to take home some books and papers I might need urgently, I thought it was worth walking in. At the time I had no idea it would be over a year before I would see my office again. Along unusually quiet city streets, I caught the eye of passers-by and saw reflected what was probably the same look on my face: *apprehension, concern, anxiety* and *disturbance*. One random woman – perhaps a little older than myself – stopped me, touched my arm and said 'my god, this is bad, what are we going to do?' Across these looks, glances, conversations in the first hours there was a sense not merely of crisis, but of a rupture from our everyday normativities; a change that felt drastic and unknowable.

Having spent a lot of time researching and writing about cultural concepts of population, which included encountering apocalyptic films, books and television series that depict radical de-population, I was aware that one lens through which I was immediately utilizing to make sense of the news, the anxiety on people's faces and the sudden shock of my campus closing down, was apocalyptic thinking. That is, through the fear that civilization, society, everyday life, comfort, the certainty of food and shelter for ordinary, middle-class Western professionals like myself are significantly more precarious than we like. Or, if following the mundane narrative of apocalyptic film and novels, that something 'alien' sweeps across the world taking away the infrastructural supports that provide safety and comfort leaving one having to manage one's own survival.

At the same time, however, being familiar with historian and theorist Michel Foucault's (2007) unpacking of the historical management of plague through lockdown, division, disciplinary and biopolitical practices of control and surveillance, the other lens available to think about this sudden change was through the knowledge that if we are careful not to spread disease, we live through the disruption without losing civilization. Measures of quarantining, dividing towns, requiring citizens to stay at home, preventing travel, are not new practices for combatting disease but, indeed, very old ones with proven track records of success. Thinking about such measures of the past and how they were beginning to unfold contemporaneously in those early COVID days was, naturally, clouded with concerns about how such measures are so often unevenly distributed, undemocratically experienced and unavailable to some while protective of others. Across both of these lenses, however, as I walked to my office, was that no matter whether COVID-19 was to be read as a moment of apocalypse or a moment of careful, well-planned survival, the rupture to everydayness *must* have an impact on how our identities are constituted in the peaceful banality of everyday movement, connection, temporal flows of work-and-home, social belonging and perceptions of inviolability to disease.

Writing nearly three years on from that day, it is much easier to unpack some of the ways in which the COVID-19 pandemic has had that anticipated impact on identity, belonging and social participation, including the ways in which its representation as a crisis or rupture of everydayness performed a re-constitutive force on subjectivity, identity and sociality. This temporal distance from the beginning of the pandemic has meant opportunities to gather evidence, including from commissioned evaluations of government COVIDSafe communication strategies I have led, digital ethnographies in online spaces discussing the pandemic health interventions, as well as the vast array of everyday media, online discourse and conversations that have dominated social and media engagement over the past three years. In some ways, these have revealed substantial surprises, such as the fact that the pandemic did not jolt the wider public into a wholesale shift towards mutual care practices. In other ways, this vast evidence confirmed some of the initial thinking that circulated in the first weeks: that the pandemic would disrupt everyday practices, how we work, how we value travel and movement, and ultimately our identities in contexts of belonging and relationality.

This book explores how our identities, beliefs, behaviours and forms of belonging are transformed by the rupture and longevity of the pandemic. Across this, and the following chapters I explore that change from a series of different angles, including the role of media discourses, the advent of mask-wearing in Western regions, the profound disruption to everyday movement brought about by lockdowns, travel and border restrictions, how we shift our ordinary use of our bodies in touch, and the advent of vaccination and anti-vaccination discourses as part of our everyday ways of responding to the pandemic. At the heart of all of these different approaches is, however, the idea of the pandemic as a crisis or rupture, possibly the most substantial occurring globally since the end of the Second World War.

In the remainder of this introduction, I would like to explore two of the key themes or 'master narratives' of the broad cultural response to COVID-19 – the formation of shock, disruption and rupture through crisis discourses, and the stories of personal resilience that have been told and circulated throughout the COVID years. These are not, of course, the only master narratives of the COVID response; rather we also have 'rejection and disbelief' which I discuss in the context of disinformation and conspiracy in the next chapter, and 'apocalyptic thinking' which I discuss in Chapter 2. I would also like to give a brief outline here as to how identity is re-constituted in the context of the combination of these competing discourses of COVID responsiveness and cultural re-framing. I will provide at the end of the chapter a break-down of some of the following chapters and approaches that address the roles of mask-wearing, restrictions on mobility, touch and isolation as the everyday experience of disruption, and their impact on how we perform our identities and sense of belonging.

Rupture: Disrupting everyday subjectivity

By early March of 2020, the reality that the world was at significant risk of a highly infectious, life-threatening and never-before-seen coronavirus was beginning to be recognized in many parts of the world as a sudden rupture to everyday life. Although the World Health Organization announced a global health emergency as early as January 2020, news that all parts of the world were facing a pandemic of proportions not witnessed in living memory circulated with substantially greater news and social media attention in March, prompting responses that can be understood as producing discontinuities with everydayness and, therefore, normative practices of identity, belonging, relationality and being. Governments in many countries responded in different ways, with some announcing urgent social distancing, bans on gatherings, closure of non-essential businesses and services, lockdowns of the population in private homes, border closures and quarantine measures.

In many cases, bio-hazard and bio-security statutory provisions were enacted and policing measures to enforce compliance were expanded. Over the first year, responses to the various measures were mixed, including protests of lockdown and curfew measures and substantial support for governments that took action. Conspiracy theories about the origin of the virus or government interventions in several Western nations circulated, while simultaneously there was a substantial increase in public interest in fact-checking, factual information and medical knowledge. Debates about measures, government and private responses in all parts of the world have continued, particularly in the context of politics, health knowledge, impact on families and work, economic theory, histories of plagues and histories of economic depression. Engagement with knowledge, debate and discourse on these topics has undoubtedly had an impact on how people everywhere view their world, particularly those who are less likely to be exposed to the actual health realities of infection or mortality.

What matters, of course, is that the *interruption* to temporal flows of everydayness brought by the response to the pandemic has been experienced in diverse ways in different parts of the globe, and experienced differently depending on socio-economic, urban/rural and gender demarcations in local settings. However, if we are to understand the experience of the disruption at an ontological level, then it is necessary also to make sense of the aspects of that experience that have been shared, which includes the interruption to a normative *everyday* stability of movement, labour, consumption, social engagement and – indeed – banal routine. I am arguing here that regardless of geographic or social setting, rupture to everydayness itself has occurred for such large numbers of people in ways which have a fundamental impact on the human condition in the twenty-first century. Such a destabilization in the normative and everyday cultural practices – which in some ways include aspects that may constitute a permanent break from normativities of the past – have significant ramifications for how we relate to each other, engage with our senses of self and how we conceive ethical obligations of care for the self and others as part of a global population (Cover 2020a).

In the early weeks after COVID-19 was declared a pandemic (World Health Organization 2020a), when restrictions on mobility and border crossings became suddenly the normative requirement of social participation in many jurisdictions (and the interruption to ordinary flows of movement, travel plans, holidays, and so on), and news and public sphere discourse became dominated by COVID-19 reports, we witnessed two frames of discourse in relation to the rupture of the norm: one suggesting that this was a short-term passing phase which will be followed by a return to normal, and the other being that what is recognizably normal is gone forever – a radical change to futurity. In terms of the first, we initially would hear people say 'this will be over before we know it', or 'soon, we'll be saying "do you remember the coronavirus" just as we said "do you remember the Swine Flu"' (e.g. Jenkins 2020), indicating an absence of crisis that will not, on the whole, disrupt normative everyday life. That is, the first frame disavows a crisis or disruption at all.

Normative continuity, however, has been invoked in other ways that see the COVID-19 pandemic as meaningful but demanding a minimization of disruption. That is, COVID-19 is a disruption not because there is a serious virus in circulation, but because governments and leaders have *over-reacted* by disrupting everyday life. This response was witnessed, for example, in placards at protests in several cities in North American and Europe demanding a 'return to normal' by ending social distancing measures or mobility restrictions (BBC 2020), typically expressing the assumption that despite the risk of SAR-CoV-2, the virus has little difference from an ordinary, *familiar* heavy season of 'the flu' (Ornstein 2020). Politicians such as former US President Donald Trump would speak of 'business as usual' (Borger 2020) while demands have come, often from the political right, to protect economies by prioritizing normal commerce that depends on everyday mobility, labour and consumption over measures to prevent the spread of the virus (Milligan 2020).

The second frame involves a discourse in which COVID-19 was perceived to produce a radical change to everydayness – a *permanent* disruption. In analysing the relationship between COVID-19 and economic structures that govern normativities, Simon Mair (2020) suggested in late March of the first year of the pandemic that there were four possible future scenarios that would emerge from the pandemic in ways which make a radical break with a current everyday social, financial, economic and labour frameworks: a socio-political and economic shift towards state-based capitalism; an alternative shift of the same to state-based socialism; a move towards a mutual aid culture that places the protection of life at the centre of economic activity; or, in the most apocalyptic of scenarios, a move towards barbarism and the breakdown of social, political and economic infrastructure.

In each of these, a radical reframing of how we live in a socio-economic sense is offered, although the reality nearly three years on is that most aspects of jurisdictional and international economic governance have remained intact. The anxieties of radical change that circulated in the early weeks of the pandemic are, perhaps, best exemplified by a *New York Times* article titled 'How to Prepare Now for the Complete End of the World' (Bowles 2020), which offered an image of flight from cities, civilizational collapse and pandemic survivors learning to live off the land. With such stories – and the unexpressed thoughts of this nature many have later confessed to having had – it is not surprising that the early months of the pandemic were perceived in terms of disruption (the second frame) or in terms of not wanting to confront that possibility, the disavowal (the first frame).

In that sense, the cultural rupture is experienced as 'crisis' not in terms of protecting the biopolitical futurity of population health in jurisdictions or more globally (Lemke 2011), but as the disruption to the everyday ways in which identities are performed and expressed through movement, social engagement, labour and consumption that disrupts everydayness, and the discourse of rupture is accompanied either by stories of overcoming and restoration of the norm, or by stories of substantial and permanent change. At the core, however, is the loss (through restriction and change) of the normativity of 'everyday' cultural formations, activities, practices and behaviours. This loss of the everydayness is marked partly by substantial adjustments to working practices for large numbers of middle-class, office and professional workers (such as working from home), job losses (especially for those who have never before experienced unemployment), shifts in everyday routines (home-schooling, changes to grocery shopping, curfews, closures of gyms and other sites of exercise), new fears about touching or being in the presence of other human bodies, anxieties about economic recovery or maintaining labour or business profitability, the unknowability of any return at this stage to a sense of 'normality' around shopping or entertainment routines and, perhaps most markedly, the radical restriction on mobility. It is a disruption to the *temporal* flow of everydayness, what we can consider the chrononormativity of lived reality through time and movement through space (Sharma 2013, 2014), for which the norm is almost always a white, middle-class framing of everyday routines and expectations around movement, work, domestic time, holidays, and so on. That is, the way in which bodies move and operate in temporal arrangements and local/global mobilities as rights, desires, aspirations and norms is radically disrupted in such a way as to disrupt our relationship with space, selfhood and relationality.

This rupture of the norm can be understood in cultural and discursive terms through the concept of *crisis*. The *pandemic as crisis* (for economy, governance, persons, health infrastructure, etc.) has been the ordinary, everyday parlance by which the disruption has been framed. Crises that shift how we perceive ourselves and our practices of social engagement are not, of course, new. Rather, much of the twenty-first century has been marked by various crises that produce new arrangements of politics, economy, lifestyle, labour and culture (e.g. the contemporary populism, disinformation and electoral crises in the United States that respond to the crisis of de-industrialization in parts leading to deprivation and disenfranchisement). For Antonio Gramsci (1971: 179), socio-political organic crises emerge in ways which demonstrate to the public that 'uncurable structural contradictions have revealed themselves'. The COVID-19 pandemic crisis, of course, reveals not only some of the infrastructural unpreparedness in many jurisdictions for coping with mass illness, but also the overwhelming *reliance* on the flow of everyday normativity, mobility, labour and social engagement that can be perceived, then, as a weakness – an inherent, subjective difficulty dealing with the out-of-the-ordinary disruption.

This is not merely because the changes to liveability caused by measures to prevent the spread of the virus are profound, but resulting from the temporal *suddenness* that is arguably more upsetting to normativity than the slower unfolding of other kinds of crisis. Chrononormativities describe the role played by perceptions of time and temporality in producing conformities and truths. They are a particularly powerful node in the constitution of identities which not only draw on cultural norms but also stabilize alongside the longevity of those norms which, themselves, become stereotypes over time and about the place of the self in time. What is significant about the relationship between time and normativity is that norms come to be norms because they have stabilized *over time* in such a way as to remove their historical specificity. While the slow unfolding of change makes it difficult to apprehend the ongoing cultural evolution of a norm, a sudden rupture not only draws attention to role of temporality in normativity but allows a shift to be represented as the end of one norm and the potential unknowability as to whether or not another will replace it.

Stuart Hall (1979) argued that, rather than being understood as a rupture that destroys the past, crises are *formative*. He described such productive formation in response to crises this way: 'a new balance of forces, the emergence of new elements, ... new political configurations and "philosophies", a profound restructuring of ... ideological discourses ... pointing to a new result, a new sort of "settlement" – "within certain limits'" (15). Although intended to describe the operations of populist power blocs, this also quite nicely describes the way in which the *sudden* shift in our everydayness brought about by the COVID-19 pandemic perceived as a crisis produces the space for the emergence of a new set of practices for identity, liveability, mobility and belonging: unknowable and unforeseeable, operating in the liminality of radical change in process.

Suddenness drives the representation of the pandemic not as remarkable or novel but as crisis itself. Liminality, defined as the quality of ambiguity of being located physically, emotionally, culturally or in terms of identity in a space or time of threshold (Turner 1969), is a useful way of framing the contemporary situation of COVID-19 as a disruption, rupture or crisis, particularly in terms of the unknowability in the early months as to whether a vaccine would be possible, as to how the virus would vary or mutate, or in terms of the (still unknown) longer-term impact of a virus on otherwise healthy bodies. At the same time, of course, those jurisdictions that experienced lockdowns often could not know in advance for how long, the effect on the consistency of employment or the length of bans on international travel . The latter included in some cases those who were unable to return to their home countries. In all cases, unknowability becomes the affectively felt and anxiety-provoking sense of being in the liminal space of crisis and disruption. And this, as I discuss in later chapters, has a profound effect in re-constituting our practices of identity and social belonging.

This sense of unknowability in disruption is, for Maurizio Lazzarato (2013), an aporia, since rupture emerges both from within history and from that which is outside history (20). In the context of COVID-19, it is arguable that the massive disruption to the everyday was simultaneously foreseeable and unforeseeable. The normative mobility of human bodies through global travel and tourism – constituting one of the largest industries in the world and accounting for at least '8.7 per cent of world employment and 10.3 per cent of world GDP' (Urry 2007: 4) – effectively predicts the spread of disease among human populations. At the same time, the unprecedented scale and virulence of SARS-CoV-2, its 'alienness' to human life as a virus found previously only in animals, and its impact on populations, economies and mobility beyond any other disease in living memory makes it simultaneously that which emerges from both *within* and *outside* of the unfolding of cultural history. This is how *crisis* comes to be *cultural rupture*. While Lazzarato (2013) rightly sees 'crisis' as a *permanent* mode of contemporary Western and international politics and history since at least the 1970s, an active cultural product designed to enable neoliberal and biopolitical governance (10), the crisis operates as a *transformative rupture* through that aporia of seen and unseen, knowable and unknowable (Duggan 2003: 87). The form that transformation takes is, then, not something that can be mapped in advance, opening a further space of liminality in which subjectivity loses its ground.

The convergence of the concepts of crisis, unknowability, liminality, disruption and cultural rupture marked social life and liveability through the years of the COVID-19 pandemic. It is a prevailing 'master narrative' providing 'us' with the cues for a response that is grounded in shock, anxiety, discomfort and uncertainty. However, referring to an 'us' should never be read as suggesting that everyone experienced the onset of the COVID years in the same way, or that the anxiety and discomfort were evenly shared. As corporeal, embodied subjects cohabiting a world of interdependency we do, of course, share aspects of vulnerability to this virus. However, that does not mean that we share the experience of risk, precarity, the experience of mandatory measures to prevent the virus' spread or the access to life-saving health infrastructures (Berlant 2016).

I return to this framework of cultural rupture, unevenly experience, throughout this book by assessing it from the perspective of discrete topical 'issues' that emerged during the first three years of the pandemic. These include particularly the rupture to everyday practices of mobility, to exposure to breath and air in the introduction of mask-wearing in parts of the world where this has been uncommon, the changes to formations of touch in the context of social distancing and the shifts in a normative sense of futurity. All of these are cultural elements that frame or serve as norms for performative identity, marking our ways of belonging in intelligible, coherent and relational ways. While changing practices is an ordinary part of cultural emergence and social change, the suddenness of change, the mandating of forbidden and necessary acts, and the shifts in temporal expectations all impinge upon the norms of identity that make us appear intelligible subjects in the face of others.

Resilience: Individual or in interdependency?

While disruption, rupture and radical change presented one master narrative governing the frames of discourse for the COVID years, there has also been a competing narrative and practice of storytelling: stories of resilience (in two registers). Indeed, discussions of resilience have been given significant attention from the very early months of COVID-19 before the virus was genuinely global, and these have included stories of personal survival, stories of hope in how economies or infrastructure will 'bounce back' and – somewhat conversely – stories of mutual care and support in social belonging. The concept of resilience is an awkward one to deploy in trying to understand the social frameworks of COVID-related storytelling, as there are two very different understandings of resilience, one which perceives resilience as the personal trait of an individual, and another which is more interested in how resilience is fostered within social engagement.

Developed by Crawford Holling in the 1970s, the concept of resilience was originally used to describe the capacity of a system to 'absorb change and disturbance and still maintain the same relationships between populations or state variables' (Holling 1973: 14). In terms of ecology and the physical sciences, the notion of resilience works within an assumption that future events will not be known or expected, thereby requiring a capacity to accommodate those events whatever form they take (21). The first approach in relation to human subjects occurred in the psychological sciences, where the term was deployed to make sense of a subject's capacity to 'bounce back' from adverse life events and adapt to new situations or changed conditions. The difficulty with the psychological approach is the tendency to presume a unitary, independent subject for whom resilience is experienced personally and in a unitary way (Leipold and Greve 2009). Here, resilience is typically considered an innate quality, used as a factor to explain why some subjects overcome adverse conditions or vulnerabilities while others fail.

Such psychological approaches to resilience are arguably unhelpful, since no subject exists in a way divorced from social engagement, interactions, mutually supportive infrastructures, or shared languages and discourses. This is a key point I emphasize throughout this book. The alternative approach is known as the 'social ecology of resilience' (Unger 2012a), and understands the source of resilience to be experienced primarily in terms of the physical, social and emotional environment inhabited by a human subject. In this context, resilience can be understood as

> a set of behaviors over time that reflect the interactions between individuals and their environments, in particular the opportunities for personal growth that are available and accessible... The likelihood that these interactions will

promote well-being under adversity depends on the meaningfulness of these opportunities and the quality of the resources provided .... [R]esilience results from a cluster of ecological factors that predict positive human development (more that individual traits), and that the effect of an individual's capacity to cope and the resources he or she has is influenced by the nature of the challenges the individual faces.

(Unger 2012b: 14)

Resilience here is interactional rather than a personal 'asset'; it is a shared quality by which individuals recover and sustain liveability against threats through engagement with and by communities, cultures, families, populations and institutions. A social ecology approach to resilience understands it therefore as more than self-efficacy, self-esteem, attachment or other protective factors but, instead, as the 'complex interactive processes embedded in social and physical ecologies that contain levels of risk that exceed the norm' (Unger 2012b: 27).

Both conceptual versions of resilience form many of the stories of the experience of the pandemic across the years since its beginning. On the one hand, we have guidance on resilience provided in the context of managing mental health that primarily emphasize individual capabilities. For example, the Uniting Church in Australia provided online guidance comprised of six activities to manage mental health and resilience during lockdown periods: staying active through yoga; walking the dog or dancing to music at home; eating well; getting good sleep; staying hydrated; relaxing through breathing exercises or gardening; and talking to others on the phone if feeling stressed (Uniting NSW 2020). The first five are primarily physiological and individualistic, and only the last involves drawing on the peer-support of a network that acknowledges the interdependency of social life.

When we consider the social-ecological approach, however, we see stories that emphasize interaction between people in interdependency as the starting point of resilience. Perhaps the most prominent example in the early weeks of the pandemic as it was experienced in Italy was the trend in which people in apartment blocks and streets would sing together from balconies while quarantined. Often described as an outpouring of 'solidarity' (Thorpe 2020), here the story is one of togetherness, mutual support and recognition that the disruption of COVID is not something done to individuals, but experienced socially and in interdependency. Indeed, juxtaposing the two different registers by which resilience has been discussed in the COVID years – individualistic trait or dependent on social networks – is a core consideration in this book. While much of the disinformation, anti-vaxxer, protest and disavowal discourses draw on a liberal-humanist individualism and a myth of human independency, we are reminded by *both* the spread of the virus and the stories of resilience, care and mutual support of the way in which human identity is grounded in a shared interdependency.

Philosopher Judith Butler (2020) argues for a need to counter individualism and myths of masculine-independent survival, and embrace the *a priori* fact of interdependency as a foundational aspect of human subjectivity. She argues that 'no body can sustain itself on its own' but that all corporeal life is constituted precisely in 'its lack of self-sufficiency' (49). This interdependency is infused in our everyday embodied lives from corporeal support to social relations, psychic dependency on relationalities, the infrastructures that enable movement and mobility, and the tools that enable communication. This constitutive interdependency grounds the kinds of supportive, ecological resiliencies that are told in some of the COVID stories. At the same time, however, our constitutive interdependency is a factor in what enables COVID-19 to spread in the first place: the fact our bodies come together, socially, connectively and in ways which enable an aerosolized virus to spread from orifice to orifice on a global scale means the unavoidable *fact* of our identities as social makes it difficult to avoid the risks that interdependency carries. I will return to the centrality of interdependency as constitutive of our human identities and practices of belonging several times over the next chapters.

COVID stories and identity

The two master narratives presented above – COVID as radical rupture and COVID experiences of resilience whether individualist or interdependent – provide the core cultural and communicative frameworks by which our identities are formed and re-formed through the crisis of the pandemic. As I discuss in later chapters, if we understand identity, subjectivity and selfhood to be constituted in language encountered through available discourses, the overriding discourses of COVID not only re-frame how we think about the world, but how we experience ourselves as identities in that world. COVID changes how we perform ourselves, whether that's the corporeal response to social distancing requirements, the semi-conscious stepping away from a person who is coughing, the change in routines that isolation and then post-isolation causes, the obscuring of the face as the marker of identity once mask-wearing became normative, the way we react to others who are obeying or disobeying mandatory safety measures, the way our perception of space changes when travel beyond the local shop is forbidden and what it means to spend every hour with a partner, children or a housemate when a life had previously been built on spending hours each day separated.

To make sense of the impact of COVID stories, media discourses and safety practices on our identities, social participation and practices of belonging, I will take these narratives to task across short chapters in this book. The first two chapters of this book explore the significance of media and public discourses about COVID-19 – that is, the linguistic, cultural and media settings that make available the discourses through which we perceive and perform our identities, behaviours and forms of social belonging. Focusing on media and communication, the next chapter explores some of the competing media discourses of the COVID-19 pandemic, from health advisory material to the role of disinformation and dissent, and the disjuncture between them that called upon audience to do the 'hard work' of making sense of our changed social and global world. Considering the role of audience reception, interactivity and the making available and unavailable of various health discourses, it sets the scene for how we engage with narratives of COVID-19 in English-speaking regions. This is followed by a chapter exploring how apocalyptic fictions, stories and films played a substantial role in providing one particular framework which 'cued' the hopelessness response; I suggest there that some of the ways in which interdependency are civilization are perceived as threatened, vulnerable and precarious in apocalyptic stories conditioned how identities are re-framed as threatened.

Chapter 3 launches the theoretical exploration of how these various, competing discourses are drawn upon in the context of 'crisis' and 'disruption' in producing change, reconstitution and re-framing of identity and selfhood during the pandemic. Drawing on Judith Butler's theories of performativity, the chapter presents an account for how cultural rupture can be understood to affect selfhood and subjectivity, whereby a breach in normative everydayness prompts the re-constitution of subjectivity itself. The chapter explores how the reconfiguration of identity is experienced as corporeal and as a site of anxiety and destabilization of the self, calling upon subjects to renew or re-stabilize identity.

Chapters 4–6 investigate 'disruption' to everydayness across a range of different frameworks and COVID-19 experiences. Chapter 4 asks what happens to identity when mobility – a taken-for-granted right among some (not all) of a freedom to move about towns, regions, cities, crossing borders, at will and leisure – is substantially restricted in the jurisdictions where lockdowns, quarantining and other constraints on movement occurred. Chapter 5 considers how masks and the changes to practices of being face-to-face have an impact on how we perform and perceive our identities as visual and corporeal subjects. This includes our changing relationship with space and distance, our perception of spaces that are normatively busy but suddenly deathly quiet, and the way in which this has been represented in images. Chapter 6 considers other corporeal practices that changed as a result of the pandemic – this time in the context of social distancing and the reduced capacity for people to touch one another. Touch is a central part of social engagement, whether a handshake, a hug or casually bumping a stranger in the street. Drawing on Elizabeth Grosz' work on spaces and corporeal assemblages, the chapter accounts for how the body *as* subjectivity was radically disrupted by sudden changes in practices of touch, physicality and intimacy.

Chapter 7 investigates another important angle in assessing how discourses of disruption, health, media and disinformation play into aspects related to identity and a sense of vulnerability: vaccination and anti-vaxxer beliefs. Vaccination has variously been discussed in public settings as either a magic bullet that will end the pandemic (when a certain percentage of vaccinated population is reached), perceived as a lie (conspiracy theories that vaccination is a trick to insert a tracking chip in human bodies) and through a discourse of risk management and risk awareness, in which different vaccines are 'weighed up' by individuals in making choices about vaccination. Key here is the extension of twentieth- and twenty-first-century biopolitical practices of risk 'calculation' further into the site of personal and social health. Chapter 8 considers the role of temporality and social change, considering some of the ways in which a failure to mourn the lost practices of the past resulted in not only increased anxiety but disavowal of the realities of the pandemic. I conclude this work with a short discussion that looks to a normative post-COVID world in which high rates of infection and death continue, and in which (at the time of writing) those political leaders who have announced the end of the pandemic have spoken too soon. Significant here is weighing up some of the possibilities of a more ethical way of being ethical through equitable social interdependency through what has been learned from the disruption of the pandemic.

1

Media discourses of coronavirus: From health advisory to conspiracy

Introduction

In the previous introduction, I presented some of the ways in which two core stories or 'master narratives' about human life, identity, survival and behaviour have circulated as responses to the onset of the COVID-19 pandemic: recognizing the pandemic as crisis in ways which are perceived as a disruption of everyday norms that condition our identities, and stories of resilience – whether individualistic or based in mutual care and social support – that describe survival and shared conditions of interdependency. Another way in which we can make sense of the significance of narrative, discourse and information in the context of the pandemic, and how these inflect our identities as human beings confronted with a serious, life-threatening virus, is through the range of media and information discourses available to us.

The COVID-19 pandemic has probably involved one of the most extensive sets of media stories in recorded history. Towards the end of the first year of the pandemic, *The Economist* (2020) noted that only the First and Second World Wars were events resulting in greater news coverage. Given the extent to which news circulates today – as opposed to the period of the end of the Second World War, where it was limited to radio, print and film – it is not unreasonable to suggest that the amount of words written, voices disseminated and videos recorded has been greater than any other major past global event. What this means for people across the world, then, is that there has been an overwhelming rate and distribution of information and discourse, vast discussion, as well as substantial conflicting viewpoints and opinions on the virus, infection prevention measures, the development and distribution of vaccines, the shift from prevention to 'COVID Normal' behaviours, perceptions that the pandemic has ended, and beliefs and attitudes about the future of population health.

Although there are, of course, some who will have turned away from news, media and platform discourse about the pandemic to avoid the ill-effects of what has sometimes been referred to as 'doom-scrolling' (Mannell and Meese 2022), the majority of people across the planet with access to broadcast and digital media have been exposed to significantly high rates of complex information, disinformation and other media storytelling about the pandemic. We already know that exposure and engagement with any media form and the discourses that various media and platforms make available have a substantial impact on the performativity of identity, the shaping of attitude and behaviour, and on the perception of belonging and non-belonging (Cover 2016). Putting that exposure and engagement into the context of massive media coverage and online debate during a crisis or culturally disruptive instance of a protracted pandemic can do nothing but reframe the media-identity relationship in ways which change who we are.

One factor that was widely experienced in urban western regions throughout the pandemic has been an increase in what is often referred to as 'screen time' – more time engaging with broadcast news, absorbing and sharing information found on websites and social media, and practising our social engagement across platforms. Workplaces shifted from norms of in-person meetings to bringing people together by video-conferencing, students were taught across Zoom, conferences were cancelled in favour of sharing recorded material, and families separated by travel restrictions took up the affordances of digital technologies to spend time with one another in ways previously unfamiliar or less common. The additional screen time that, for many, replaced outdoor activities, social activities and other face-to-face engagement has contributed to the additional exposure to competing media discourses about COVID-19.

To make sense of the role media and communication have played in the shifts and reframings of identity practices during the COVID years, I will begin with a brief summary of the broad pandemic-related discourses that have dominated media and communication, followed by some analysis of what it means to engage with health communication and information. I follow this with a discussion of the important factor of fake news, disinformation and misinformation which has been a key controversy in COVID-related information, before addressing some of the ways in which we can apprehend the roles of digital interactivity, participation and polarization in producing a fractured approach to pandemic discourses. I end this chapter by assessing the ways in which we need to recognize the significance of practices of audience reception (as opposed to linear understandings of communication) if we are to make sense of the role media plays in shaping identities in the era of a pandemic.

Media content about the pandemic

I do not want to spend time in this chapter providing a full assessment of the global media and digital communication content about COVID-19 – a phenomenal task given the vast amount of material that has circulated, as well as the substantial COVID-related disinformation and misinformation that circulated but has judiciously been made unavailable. Rather, if we are to make sense of how COVID-related information, knowledge and media have an impact on how we perceive our identities, it is not the *content* that matters, but the *cultural practices of engaging* with media that needs to be unpacked. With that in mind, it is more useful to begin with some thoughts about the broad strokes of media coverage, including particularly the principal discourses that govern the kinds of information and content disseminated with which we have interacted.

We could say here that there have been four media and communication discourses in contemporary public sphere dialogue about the pandemic that matter for thinking about identity in the COVID years. Firstly, there has been a *biopolitical dialogue* that looks to the figure of 'population' in terms of numbers, statistics, normative distributions, impact of the virus on different age-groups, border closures, implications for migrant populations, vaccination programmes and hospital capacities (Cover 2020a). Biopolitics involves the administrative attempt to modify aspects of discipline for use in broader-scale governance (Foucault 2004a: 242). While biopolitics is a normative function of governance and administration focused on the politicization of life itself (Lemke 2011: 3), it becomes a point of intent and interest in public sphere discourse in various waves, usually when the idea of population re-emerges as a political, cultural or social issue. In the case of the pandemic, we have witnessed a substantial form of reporting that draws on biopolitical language that for Foucault (2007) finds one strand of its origins in the discourse around smallpox:

> [H]ow many people are infected with smallpox, at what age, with what effects, with what mortality rate, lesions or after-effects, the risks of inoculation, the probability of an individual dying or being infected by smallpox despite inoculation, and the statistical effects on the population in general.

(11)

Biopolitics is a practice that shapes the liveability not of individual lives (managed through institutions and disciplinary practices) but of whole populations, regulating behaviours through a combination of measurements and requirements that seek 'an equilibrium, maintain an average, establish a sort of homeostasis, and compensate for variations within this general population and its aleatory field' (Foucault 2004a: 246). In a media-saturated world, of course, part of those regulatory practices are deployed through media not by the announcement of restrictions but by the circulation of norms. These are not the norms articulated by disciplinary institutions (schools, health authorities, etc.) that prescribe a dichotomy of 'normal' and 'abnormal' behaviours. Rather, in a biopolitical knowledge framework, behaviours, health and attitudes are plotted along a less-restrictive but equally powerful 'distributional curve' of normativities (Foucault 2007: 63). The extent to which one complies with such regulatory practices is driven not merely by governmental instructions but by how one perceives the norms at play through media coverage of the extent to which others are non-compliant. Whether one checks-in diligently when entering a place of business in jurisdictions which mandated such tracking, or occasionally skips it depends on compliance data circulating in the press that describes the distribution of normative compliance.

One substantial, daily aspect of many news media services was a biopolitical framework of reporting. For example, online newspaper banners carrying updates on statistics of infection, death rates, compliance, vaccination rates, and so on. Many online and television news services gave COVID-19 statistics in the familiar format of weather reports and stock exchange news. In each case, and drawing on data derived from local health departments, the World Health Organization, the Centres for Disease Control, among others, what is communicated ostensibly to inform the public simultaneously serves as a knowledge framework against which we are invited to plot our own health, survival, practices, timing of vaccination and safety to move about or be less diligent in wearing a mask – sometimes regardless of formal health recommendations or mandatory measures. Such shaping constitutes not merely how we behave in a pandemic, but who we are.

A second media discourse during the pandemic contrasted significantly with the biopolitical by drawing not on population concepts that frame the pandemic in terms of overall health a wide group of people and thereby set curves of normativities against which to plot one's own behaviour, sense of self or belonging. This second discourse is, rather, a more individualistic and liberalistic framework that is both disciplinary and interested not in the preservation of the life of whole populations but the conduct of people (Macey 2009). This is witnessed in news reports, social media discussions, official and informal advice on how individuals (and families) can, should or currently are navigating liveability through lockdowns, stories on where it is safe for a person to go, how to stay fit when working from home or guidance on the home-schooling of children, and so on. It incorporates many of the individual resilience stories described in the introduction, as guidance on how to live during disrupted circumstances.

A prominent story in this framework in the early years of the pandemic was one which described people's individual experience of contracting COVID-19, particularly the early viral strains including 'Delta'. This was a significant kind of story, contrasting not only with the wider population health and biopolitical frame, but with the health advisory information that circulated describing anticipated symptoms in clinical terms. Stories such as this often drew on and repeated people's individual social media posts, relating people's experience of the onset of symptoms and the order in which some experienced them – mild nausea, fever, nasal congestion, sore throat and mild cough (Forsey 2020). Placing the symptoms into the lived experience of individuals through drawing on their own storytelling here allowed a different kind of response to media content: the ability to measure, contrast and compare, assess potential symptoms and gain a knowledge capability on the virus and its effects without needing to rely on official information which often did not articulate distinctions between ages (other than that the elderly were at greater risk) or provide stories of recovery against which those affected could measure their own progress.

Thirdly, there has been a discourse that relates to expressions of vulnerability and precarity, drawing on elements of both the biopolitical and liberalistic perspectives outlined above. Vulnerability, as we know from Butler (2004), is a shared condition of human subjectivity which is constituted from the very beginning in the embodied need for mutual care and dependency on the social for life itself. That shared experience of primary vulnerability is, however, hidden by interpretative frames which figure subjects' 'worthiness of protection' differentially in ways which allow some lives to be fostered and some to be disregarded (Butler 2009: 50).

We see stories of vulnerability primarily in media reporting on the differential impact of COVID-19 on people. A prominent narrative has related to front-line health workers, including particularly relating examples in which medical and ambulance staff have 'burned out' during the excess workload of dealing with spikes in infections (Cunningham 2022), although vulnerability is also often a frame discussing COVID-19 in relation to homeless persons around the world (Booker 2021). While the shared experience of a struggle against a pandemic *might* have invoked the shared experience of bodily precarity, the reality has been that the discursive frames that differentiate between worthy and unworthy lives have remained in place, such that various articulations about vulnerability tend to be particular and dichotomized (various groups suffering job losses while others do not), tendencies towards nationalist claims (such as around access to vaccines over shared responsibility for the globe) and the galvanization of claims to vulnerability in certain conspiracy theories (such as that some populations are seen to be vulnerable to manipulation by a 'deep state' supposedly working for a supposed liberal elite). Here, crisis and rupture are figured as moments demanding redress, even if those claims to redress about by those already benefitting from extant socio-economic structures.

Finally, there has been an antagonistic discourse that is broadly liberal-humanist and individualist, grounded in a radical disavowal of governmental health measures, restrictions, the efficacy of vaccination, mandatory mask-wearing or social distancing, and so on. This discourse is based partly in the kinds of disinformation I discuss below, and partly in a wider populism that represents 'everyday' people's needs or desires as being ignored by a political elite whose activities, decisions and legislative practices are deemed to be untrustworthy or conspiratorial (Cover 2020b). These are often narratives relating the reasons why people have attended anti-lockdown protests or anti-vaccination rallies (Paynter 2020). Here, stories justifying an emotive response to the conditions of regulatory health measures have been a significant aspect of this media discourse – why people are angry, upset, anxious, often including interview material from protesters describing why others should feel similarly. Again, certain arguments for what some consider 'normative' behaviour or attitude are articulated, calling upon readers and viewers to manage their own emotional and affective responses in the context of a large sample of such narratives during various periods of the COVID years.

Engaging with health communication

Communicating credible, scientifically based health information through media sources has long been understood as challenging (Penders et al. 2017), and it is widely recognized that while some people will draw their health information from credible, authorized, government or health authority services and websites, others rely primarily on the matrix of news, media, documentary and social media platform posts. Given the competing media discourses described above, this presents additional challenges for ensuring people can manage what we might consider here to be 'healthy identities' that incorporate everyday practices to prevent contraction and spread of the virus.

In early 2021, I led a study for the State Government of Victoria (Australia) to evaluate the effectiveness of their COVID-19 communication strategy for providing information to culturally and linguistically diverse (CALD) young people in the state. In Australia, state governments have jurisdictional responsibility for many aspects of health delivery, and were therefore heavily involved in the communication of safety measures, including adherence to social distancing rules, the importance of compliance with mask-wearing mandates, the reasons why a sustained stay-at-home lockdown was being maintained and requirements if a person in that state becomes infected or unwell. Given some government concerns that residents for whom English was not the first language may not be engaged with ordinary news services or undertake their own information-seeking, the government attempted a range of communication campaigns to encourage compliance and good health behaviours.

In the course of the study, my team and I spoke with a number of young people in the campaigns' target audience communities to understand their health-related information-seeking habits, their understanding of COVID-related health safety measures and their views on the campaigns. We found among our interviewees that, contrary to government expectations that young people do not engage with authoritative information, many younger CALD-community members regularly consumed news with substantial trust, but did not necessarily seek out further health information from, say, government websites. Indeed, a core finding of the study was that younger audience members had substantially increased their engagement with media to seek information and updates on COVID-19 and, importantly, as a mechanism that gave a sense of belonging in the wider community. What was significant here was not that our interviewees were deliberately seeking health information in order to guide their own conscious practices, but that they ritualistically engaged with an array of media from traditional news sources to social media and navigated across these as a practice of identification and social belonging with a wider population. Here, again, the content is much less important than the cultural activity.

Engaging with news services of various kinds is, indeed, one of the ways in which the resilience and belonging through practices of interdependency I described in the introduction is enabled. In his book *Communication as Culture* (1988), media theorist James Carey identified two views of communication that perceive the audience in two different ways – the *transmission* view and the *ritual* view. The transmission view is the standard, pedestrian account of communication as it occurs in most simplistic communication models of sender-message-receiver. It is, for Carey, defined by key terms such as 'imparting', 'sending', 'transmitting' and 'giving information to others'. Media content is seen in this view as distributed *across space* to audiences, whether that's a social media post or television news (14). He described the ritual view, on the other hand, as communication acts that were about 'sharing', 'association', 'fellowship' and 'possession of a common faith' among audiences. Here it was not the text itself that mattered – rather, the regular, ritualistic engagement of an audience that gives a sense of commonality, community, interdependency and being on a shared journey together. In those ritualistic practices, then, an identity is shaped and formed by the performative act of engagement rather than by the content.

Fake news and conspiracy

Fake news, disinformation and misinformation about COVID-19 were recognized as spreading quickly from the very early weeks of the identification of the virus in Wuhan, China (Depoux et al. 2020). A UK report revealed that almost half (46 per cent) of the country had been exposed to fake news about the virus within the first year of the pandemic (OfCom 2020), with similar concerns reported in the United States, including data that two-thirds of the population had seen false stories on a daily basis (Mitchell and Oliphant 2020). The World Health Organization labelled this emergent framework an 'infodemic', where *both* overwhelming credible information and large rates of misinformation substantially challenged the quality of necessary, crisis-driven health communication (World Health Organization 2020b).

In the twenty-first century, fake news can be described as follows: deceptive content circulated primarily through digital networks, created deliberately to shape a particular public viewpoint or perception of a topic. It is broadly understood as text (including audio or video) which purports to be news but is intentionally and verifiably false, aiming to mislead readers and viewers (Allcott and Gentzkow 2017: 213). It generally relies on a kind of 'trickery' whereby those deliberately circulating fake news for nefarious purposes do so by dressing up information in a form that might appear to be news (e.g. adopting the tone, style, newsworthiness and pyramiding functions of recognizable news) and with embellishments that make it appear to be from a credible news source (e.g. a website that has an address, or URL, very closely matching that of a recognized news site, or the deliberate use of banners, headers and logos of credible news sites).

The emergence of fake news, disinformation and misinformation is, of course, a separate and alarming cultural phenomenon, resulting partly from the affordances of online communication lacking editorial and gate-keeping processes, the rise of malicious state and non-state criminal actors using disinformation, and a wider populism that distrusts traditionally credible news sources (Cover, Haw and Thompson 2022). Fake news and disinformation are not simply a matter of communication becoming more complex in the twenty-first century, or a problem of the extra labour demanded of communication professionals in a twenty-four-hour news cycle to ensure factual communication, but has had a wider impact on the everyday lives of ordinary people in discerning and relying on factual content. This new phase is marked by the digital affordances that allow a group of actors to believe they can or should produce alternative content that tricks people into believing their non-evidenced perspective or shapes a readership into adhering to a particular belief or attitude. And it is the emergent conditions that make it possible for such media to be unwittingly circulated by the misinformed as become a *normative* experience of everyday life.

When a fake news story tells us, for example, that the COVID-19 virus is a weapon deliberately designed by Islamists to wipe out Western civilization (Miller 2020), it draws, on the one hand, on a longer history and cultural practice or tabloid sensationalism designed to invoke alarm, fear or anxiety and, on the other, appeals to an existing audience who have already been positioned to distrust normative political communication, to see 'the other' as a dangerous enemy, or to who are pre-prepared to feel outrage (towards Muslims or the leadership of the People's Republic of China) when they read the fake news story (Forrest, Blair and Dunn 2020). And, finally, it includes an audience segment that deliberately seeks out such stories to circulate them further (Cover, Haw and Thompson 2022) or to contribute to a comforting – albeit suspicious – world-view that transforms crisis and chaos into conspiracy; a case of what communication strategist Parnell Palme McGuiness (2021) described as the practice of those people 'who pick up an idea and knit it into a system of beliefs that becomes their whole world, to the exclusion of reality'.

Disinformation that 'fits' into a conspiracy theory – such as that the virus was deliberately manufactured, that the illness is caused by 5G mobile telephony towers or that the vaccination programme is inserting tracking chips in human bodies – has a higher likelihood of being taken on as fact during a period in which an existential need is threatened (Douglas et al. 2019: 8). That is, there is a risk that such disinformation, whatever the purpose of its original fabrication, is received by some audience members positively as a way of making sense of an anxiety-provoking crisis. This is particularly the case for those without reasonable or equitable access to genuine credible information. Those who are disenfranchised (through no fault of their own) utilize such conspiracy theories to gain a sense of agency by perceiving themselves as having accessed a 'hidden truth' behind the complex situation in which they have found themselves (Singh Grewal 2016: 26).

The substantial recognition that disinformation was a problem did, however, result in one counter-discourse that contributed to the media matrix of competing knowledge frameworks. A widespread active public condemned disinformation and the sharing of fake news stories as misinformation. The hashtag 'Covidiots' came to be widely used to call out those who were knowingly or unwittingly spreading disinformation and misleading health information. Arguably, this is not an ethical counter-discourse: ignorance is not a 'lack' for which some members of the public should be shamed or made to feel responsible; rather, it is a culturally produced disposition conditioned by education systems that disavow critical engagement with textuality (Gilson 2011), and facilitated by the transactional nature of media consumption and information overload (Papacharissi 2015: 44). These factors point to the need for a critical and cultural pedagogy to educate the public on fake news the myriad forms it takes, how to detect it and avoid spreading.

The more useful and more ethical outcome of the widespread recognition of disinformation was that attempts to explain to those who had taken up conspiracy theories and misleading content resulted in a massive and unprecedented increase in public knowledge of virology, epidemiology and genomics as they circulate in everyday communication. Indeed, it is possible to argue that the pandemic has produced a *very* substantial cultural shift in which the competing knowledge frameworks have, on the one hand, created anxieties for identity, belonging, behaviour and attitude but, on the other, have vastly increased access to health and epidemiological knowledge frameworks that *should* be better available to the public. Certainly, most of us will have significantly increased our understanding of statistics, mRNA vaccine technologies and quarantine practices over the past few years.

Digital interactivity, participation and polarization

In contrast with other serious pandemics of the past, such as the 1917 influenza pandemic, is the fact that COVID-19 has occurred in an era of participatory and interactive digital communication, rather than the past in which health communication was disseminated through traditional media that was governed by editorial gate-keeping practices. Even for the most discerning reader and consumer of credible information sources, the constant presence of social media platforms and the opportunity for everyday citizens to participate not only in storytelling but also in information creation has contributed to the complexification of knowledges about COVID-19 and to the added crisis of information credibility.

The interactivity of digital media and platform-based communication since about 2005 has resulted in several tensions in what was previously a more stable, simplified and linear process for health communication and information-sharing. By blurring the line between author and audience, eroding older technological, policy and conventional models that provided a 'control' over the text such as the printed page or the radio or television broadcast content – all of which could be said to prevent the text from being *easily* changed, adapted, re-sequenced or re-distributed, the capacity for quality information to retain its context, meaning and significance is substantially altered. This is not necessarily always a negative thing, and there is little value in taking a negative, 'blaming' or luddite approach to digital communication given it has certainly facilitated the quality of health communication and increased engagement with content. Indeed, it is important to recognize that interactive, networked media is not a 'thing' that has come and negatively changed how we *do* communication, but should be understood as the outcome of a deep-seated human desire to *participate* in storytelling, distribution or sharing (Cover 2006).

Participation in health information, then, occurs due to some changes in the 'affordances' of digital communication. This includes primarily the shift in the level of skills needed to participate in media creativity: digital skills in development, content-creation, film production and writing are no longer the province of professionally trained media practitioners (Flew 2008, Burgess and Green 2009). Rather, they became increasingly available to vast numbers capable of producing and editing their own health material – resulting in both a powerful contribution to meaning and interpretation of health information as well as the greater likelihood of disinformation. Who we are as digital selves is something which needs to be thought through the frameworks, nuances and complexities of interactivity as a theory of digital relationality, as a popular taste for engagement with stories and information that *matter* both to individuals and to a wider public.

At the same time, however, digital communication affords greater debate, adversity and argumentation, which can also result in polarized views in which people disagree so strongly they disavow *any* value of the argument or information of their opponents in an outpouring of hostility (Cover 2022). An outcome of this has been the aggressive oppositionalism between people at a time when interdependency most needs to be recognized, a contribution to the violence of protesters and a polarization between the adherents of disinformation on one side and those who struggle for quality of health communication and outcome on the other. Some of this polarized adversity over COVID-19 health communication has been blamed on the presence of online echo chambers and filter bubbles (Jiang, Ren and Ferrara 2021), although problematically, such views tend to rely on a technologically determinist perspective in which digital communication tools are incorrectly held responsible for creating the conditions for simplistic approaches to media engagement.

Echo chambers and filter bubbles, as Axel Bruns (2019) has demonstrated, are indeed possible but the anxieties about them are only warranted if a user were *only* getting *all* their information and communication from those settings. Bruns' research indicates that not only is this broadly improbable, but it is not backed up by actual evidence that people have been forced through either choice or algorithmically managed feeds to *only* engage with narrow information streams. Indeed, as Bruns shows, this kind of moral panic over echo chambers ignores the decades of genuine research that has documented the beneficial aspects of engaging with social media and other forms of online community for *expanding* the field of information and knowledge and for fostering engagement in debates that have multiple perspectives. As he notes (13), we should be wary of the ulterior motives of those who generate scepticism over social media *per se* on the misperception that social media is the source of polarization without looking to the wider cultural factors that have generated polarized views. Such factors in the case of COVID-19 include socio-economic disenfranchisement, the rhetoric of politicized populist movements and belief frameworks that precede and pre-exist the advent of the pandemic. Rather, if we are to understand this negative aspect of digital communication's impact on COVID-related behaviours, identities and practices of social belonging and adversity, then it is necessary to ask first what happens when there is a matrix of competing knowledge frameworks across media as I have described above.

Reception and engagement

To make sense of the role of media discourses about the pandemic, it is important to acknowledge that people are not simply 'duped' into believing whatever they encounter in news, information or on social media platforms. The purveyor of fake news hoaxes, Paul Horner, noted that fake news *works* precisely because in his view there is an audience who are positioned by a lack of engagement with the culture of media practices in the first place (Dewey 2016). In other words, there is nothing inherent in the practice of being a member of an audience that makes one inherently open to being misled or managed by what they encounter, whether fake news or authorized health information.

Rather, the view that anyone is unwittingly influenced or 'tricked' by any media source replicates very outdated 'media effects' models that assume media content itself universally shapes behaviours, attitudes, voting patterns and viewpoints across an inherently passive audience. Dating back to the 1930s, such approaches as the propaganda or hypodermic models of communication suggest for the greater part that the audience is not interactive with the text, does not actively interpret, analyse or create meanings around the text, and seeks no form of creative participation or redistribution of the text (Turner 1993: 206–8). Cultural studies approaches have argued for nearly half a century that audiences are empowered and active in the interpretation of meaning and the assessment of content (Radway 1988, Fiske 1989, Hall 1993), and actively use a range of tactics to interpret, resist, critique or re-utilize any text encountered (de Certeau 1984).

A more useful way of understanding the engagement with media during the COVID years is not to consider individual texts, but to recognize how different discourses (or 'ways of speaking and thinking') play an important role in forming identity, practices and behaviours, because they make available the codes of behaviour and practice that are performed reiteratively to shape our identities. Unconscious alignment of our identities and behaviours with dominant discourses makes us feel authentic and coherent as subjects (Hall 1995), and this is because such discourses are the setting that communicates the norms, categories and signifiers we are 'compelled to cite or repeat or mime' in the constitution of identity (Butler 1993: 220). An important consideration, then, is how media has not only facilitated the disseminated of certain discourses, but has made other discourses 'unavailable' that provide the resources for identity, belonging and self-positioning. This might include, for example, the kinds of discourses that provide a critical assessment of alternative ways in which to live on a planet as human beings vulnerable to disease, in favour of stories of survival and return to 'normal'. Critiques of the incursion into spaces where dangerous viruses may jump from animal to human tend to remain marginalized, thereby eschewing the opportunity to think about the interdependency between humanity and the environment we cohabit with other creatures, including dangerous viruses.

Conclusion

I have described above a range of different discourses, habits and ways of engaging with media that shed some light on how media plays a role in the cultural disruption of COVID-19 and how media discourses impinge upon our cultural practices of identity, health behaviours, social participation and belonging. What needs to be underscored in thinking about this range during a period of substantially increased media engagement and, for some, information overload (World Health Organization 2020b) is that no one is subject simply to just one media text or source on the topic, but that in a very diverse set of ways we engage with what Barbara Creed (2003) referred to as a complex 'matrix' of competing media sources that provide the terrain by which we make sense of ourselves, the world and our place in it.

When identity is performed in the context of discourses that place the cultural concepts of population and population health at the core, and the biopolitical mechanisms of statistics, distributional curves and regulatory measures are deployed and communicated, subjects are called upon to plot their identities, attitudes, behaviours and practices along those curves. Here certain distributions are considered to be 'more normal than the others, or at any rate more favorable than the others' (Foucault 2007: 63). What this means for subjectivity and identity is that in some contexts, including that of governing and caring for the self in a time of infectious disease, our actions are measured not in terms of what is 'normal' and 'abnormal' but in terms of the distance from 'the norm' along those curves. The extent to which one complies or sometimes does not comply with regulations to restrict time outdoors during mandatory lockdown periods is not a matter of compliance with those charged to police the rules but with norms communicated through media. If, for example, one travels three kilometres, but not twelve kilometres, outside of limitations from home during mandatory lockdowns, or self-diagnoses having contracted SARS-CoV-2 as a cold rather than verifying through a self-test (or the reverse), is all part of that plotting process derived from biopolitical knowledge frameworks communicated through the norms depicted in media and recognized through the behaviours of others encountered in dialogue on social media platforms.

This is an ordinary practice in the complex ways in which we perform identity, social participation and belonging. However, once we start to acknowledge how media not only make some discourses available and others unavailable, but also the complex terrain of competing knowledge frameworks, fake news, disinformation and misinformation, hyperinformation online, experiences of information overload, switching off from doom-scrolling, and so on, then the matrix of media and communication knowledge frameworks itself becomes so tense and fraught with complexities that plotting one's identity and behaviour across multiple, completing and obscure curves of normativity becomes a task marked by anxiety. Combined with the disruption and competing calls for resilience described in the introduction, the frameworks by which identity and belonging are ontologically constituted demand an even more intensive labour of self-care and preservation, beyond that which could ever be described as normative among the middle-classes in stable democracies during peace-time.

2

Apocalyptic fictions as a roadmap for crisis

Introduction

In the early days of the COVID-19 pandemic creating emergencies in the UK, the United States, Australia and New Zealand, a number of news media sources began distributing lists of pandemic-related apocalyptic film and television series (e.g. Goldsmith 2020), promoting their utility as an intertextual resource for meaning-making in a crisis situation marked by liminalities and unknowabilities. Fictional accounts – particularly film and television – provide narratives and character positionings that produce identifications (Fuss 1995) through which interpretations of factual information can be incorporated into attitude, subjectivity and behaviour (Cover 2015), and this was part of the self-conscious dissemination of apocalyptic films. Indeed, many did not need a news source suggesting apocalyptic texts. In my own case, I had previously written about apocalyptic film and television series and their role in representing the decimation of population (Cover 2020a) – like others, my thoughts in the early weeks of the pandemic turned to films such as *Contagion* (2011), *Outbreak* (1995) and series like *The Walking Dead* (2010–) as a way of gauging my own reaction and the reactions of those I saw around me.

In film and television media, global catastrophe scenarios and post-apocalyptic worlds typically present stories about a threat to the global human population from something 'alien' to a humanity that did not foresee its own vulnerability. Common examples of this alienness or otherness include, of course, a virulent disease wiping out the majority of human life on the planet, as found in, for example, *The Stand* (1994 mini-series), *Survivors* (1975 series, remade 2008–10), *12 Monkeys* (1995 film, and 2015–18 series), *Outbreak* (film), *Carriers* (2009 film) and *Contagion* (film). Many texts add a horror twist to the virus, combining it with the mythical figure of the zombie as the outcome of viral infection – these include the highly popular texts *The Walking Dead*, *28 Days Later* (2002 film), among many others.

Such narratives sit alongside and relate intertextually to screen fictions that represent other kinds of threats that cause radical depopulation and a breakdown of everyday sociality, family practices of labour and consumption, and ordinary contemporary liveability. Several of these depict the material and cultural effects of a global nuclear catastrophe, such as *Threads* (1984 film) and *The Day After* (1983 film). Others represent the cause of Armageddon through metaphors that stand in for more familiar vulnerabilities: alien invasion (*The X-Files* (1993–2002, 2016–18 series), *Falling Skies* (2011–15 series), *The Day of the Triffids* (1962 film, 1981 and 2009 series)); a meteor strike, as in *Armageddon* (1998), *Deep Impact* (1998) and *Don't Look Up* (2021); or climate change, as in *The Day After Tomorrow* (2004 film). Many of these contribute to broad cultural narratives that combine concepts of the precarity of human civilization and use disease, weapons of mass destruction and meteors as metaphors to depict other kinds of familiar 'threats' such as HIV (Shriver 2003: 155), Cold War tensions (Shaw and Youngblood 2010) and terrorism (Nikolaidis 2011).

Significant here is that the genealogy of all these films, series and in some cases the novels on which they are based has an ancestor dystopian text: Mary Shelley's (2004) novel *The Last Man*, which was published in 1826 and depicted the catastrophic end of civilization and the human population due to disease – a heritage in which illness and infection can be said to be at the core of a global melancholic attachment to civilization, its dependence on a quantum of human population and its tacit precarity. The fact that many of these texts are regularly re-made, re-booted or revived, spawning television series, comics and cross-over franchises, indicates a broad popular fascination among audiences for stories about catastrophic risk to population and global civilization, and a complex psychic attachment to these that calls for fictional stories through which to articulate concerns about loss in order to disavow the reality of everyday civilization and knowable sociality as vulnerable.

Apocalyptic stories are significant, therefore, in making sense of the cultural landscape through which COVID presented itself as a disruption to civilization and sociality, upsetting our identity-based attachment to the human population and liveability. The importance of such texts is not important because they are 'doom-oriented' or 'catastrophe-survival' stories. Rather, it is because they present an identity discourse that articulates frameworks for 'being' in ways that pivot between individual survival or resilience on the one hand, and stories about the precarity of a civilization based on population interdependency on the other.

It is possible to argue therefore that, at a deep psychic level, dystopian, catastrophic and post-apocalyptic stories of viral disease and radical population loss demonstrate a melancholic attachment to civilization: the sociality, infrastructure and cultural everydayness that give subjects a sense of relationality and belonging through stability and the 'people-ness' of place (Cover 2020a). By considering the narrative and psychic function of apocalyptic stories as cultural myths, we are well-placed to make sense of some of the cultural reactions, anxieties and sense of vulnerability that marked responses to the COVID-19 pandemic, including the counter-discourses of disavowal, denial, protest and inviolability. That is, unlike the storytelling of crisis and resilience, and unlike the media narratives of health information and disinformation, apocalyptic stories work at a deeper level by providing a roadmap not for how to behave, but for how to *feel* (or *refuse to feel*) the precarity of civil society itself.

This chapter outlines the function of the cultural narrative of disease-based apocalyptic and catastrophe storytelling in conditioning the psychic responses to real-world pandemics. I would like to consider this by addressing two aspects depicted in a representative sample of texts that represent disease-related risks of radical global de-population: firstly, the way in which such texts depict disease as a sudden radical depopulation through widespread, unexpected death – the body bags piled up in a depiction in the film *Contagion* (2011) of the outcome of a disease originating in a bat in a market in China, jumping to a pig before spreading among human beings is telling, but of course different from the 'slow death' (Berlant 2007) that accompanies the reality of disease in the contemporary world. Secondly, I investigate the way in which pandemics are depicted in these texts as something which upsets or destroys a concept of 'civilization' as contemporary life (international trade, labour, interdependency, sociality), being something based on stable human population numbers for persistence over time. What these two aspects point to is the deep-seated attachment to the world 'as we know it', whereby these stories play a cultural role of providing a space to 'contain' the anxieties over the precarity of that world and the people in it.

Apocalyptic narratives of population reduction

As I described in the previous chapter, one angle of public sphere storytelling about COVID-19 is a biopolitical one – a focus not on individuals or the individuated body-at-risk but on population numbers, flows of mobility, rates of infections, logistics of vaccine distribution and maintenance of infrastructure. In the simplest framework, 'population' means a count of people in a given space – how many people populate an area, a city, a nation-state, the world. However, it is also a socially meaningful concept that circulates across political speech, representation, the demographic and economic sciences, nationalism and racism, all in ways which govern our performance of identities through a sense of belonging (Cover 2020a). Population *numbers* are also a site of anxiety, particularly in terms of practices of exclusion of migrants (Rancière 2016), concerns over climate sustainability and over-population (Ehrlich 1968), and population loss or decimation (Shriver 2003). These competing concepts of population size, figures, make-up and knowledges are central to the ways in which subjectivity is produced and made knowable in relationality – the very thrownness of the subject into the world of a *mass of others* with whom we cohabit as a condition of being (Butler 2012: 23–4) makes the population central to the mechanisms by which identity is constituted.

When there is a concern about, or depiction of, a fundamental *shift in population numbers* such as an apocalyptic reduction of the global population to a fraction of its previously known size, the formation of population as a broadly stable, slow-changing biopolitical concept significant to identity is radically disrupted. This includes all elements that have meaning for a subject, whether kinship, place, space or recognizability. And this is what we see depicted in apocalyptic film and television where populations are radically reduced by disease or other incursion. Indeed, in the opening of Danny Boyle's *28 Days Later* (2002), we are shown the empty, globally familiar streets of London made strange and frightening by their very *failure to be populated*: he is unable to recognize either the place or himself. Similarly, the disappearance of entire populations renders all elements of a post-apocalyptic world bizarre and extraordinary.

What the post-apocalyptic depiction of survival in contemporary film and television does is demonstrate the extent to which human identity – or *humanity* itself – is constituted in a notion of stable population numbers. When those numbers are suddenly threatened (with all the implications for survival without the civilizational infrastructure based on the dispersal of skills across a population to provide electricity, food, trade, shelter and so on), human identity itself is destabilized. While population presents itself ordinarily and in normative contexts only as a backdrop or as the 'everyday' for individual subjects, its constitutive power as providing a framework for self-intelligibility only becomes apparent in those sites in which one imagines a life as a post-apocalyptic survivor in which that population is no longer present. The fear of apocalyptic scenarios of radical de-population, then, is not about a fear of the death of others, the loss of technologically derived comforts or the erasure of normative governance. Rather, it is a fear of the self becoming the unknowable – selves who are no longer recognizable to ourselves, presented with an imperative to cease everyday performativity of identity and to perform otherwise.

Some of the earlier variants of COVID-19 had a substantially high mortality rate before the introduction of the vaccines. By late 2022, there have been more than six and a half million recorded deaths attributed to the virus globally, approximately 1 per cent of infections. Sites like worldometer (www.worldometer.info) provide statistics drawn from official health department data releases across most global jurisdictions, providing infection, recovery and death rates, and – importantly – rate of cases and rate of deaths per population size for each country. Population, and its potential reduction, is thus at the heart of one aspect of COVID-19 discourse. More significantly, early media coverage took a moderate but concerning approach to anticipated mortality rates, expecting rates of 2–3 per cent (meaning approximately one death in every 30–50 people in the population), and substantially more illness (Aubusson and Cunningham 2020). At the same time, regular references in media, documentaries, referred back to other population-decimating pandemics, particularly the 1918 so-called Spanish Flu (H1N1 influenza), noting always the rate of global population death (e.g. Groch 2020), and focused not on individual stories of illness but on the impact on a global population, that is, that what may have been up to 100 million deaths did for the population of approximately 1.8 billion a century ago (Palmer 2021).

While neither the Spanish Flu nor COVID-19 produced excess mortality at rates that would threaten the overall survival of humanity, the depiction in apocalyptic films of rare, lone survivors seeking food and shelter in empty cities operates as a point of connection, exacerbated by the many media articles which listed the kinds of apocalyptic films and series to watch during the early months of COVID-19 (e.g. Sims 2020). The empty urban streets in *28 Days Later* and in series such as *The Walking Dead* or Stephen King's *The Stand* reinforce the connection as print and broadcast media accompanied articles about COVID-19 during 2020 and 2021 with images of empty city streets in regions where mandatory lockdowns were the norm. Here, the *reduction* or *absence* of the population – the peopleness of places – is the key setting of the psychic experience of anxiety about the potential mortality rate of COVID-19; not the actual outcome but the *precarity* of entire populations to disease in ways that have been unthinkable in the everyday stability and growth of the global human population.

Civilization and its vulnerabilities

Apocalyptic stories are an opportunity to play out and 'contain' our melancholic attachment to stable population by working through stories of sudden, catastrophic drops in population. The reality, of course, is that not only did the COVID-19 pandemic cause the deaths of the majority of the human population, but the filmic depiction of viral infections that kill people within hours – like insecticide on flies – is not how viral illnesses are experienced. However, what is often most pertinent in such texts' depictions is the breakdown of civilization, civil society, health infrastructure and other aspects of built environment that sustain ordinary and family liveability. Scenes of overwhelmed hospitals in *Outbreak* and *Contagion*, portrayals of shops overrun by panicking people in *The Stand*, depictions of irrational fighting in the streets or economic breakdown caused by leaders not acting quickly to secure national and state economies – these more neatly describe the precarity of our identity-based attachment not only to population, but also to the civilization, infrastructure and exchange that depend on there being a population to administer and facilitate it.

Post-apocalyptic film and television regularly centre on the connection between identity and something considered to be 'civilization' by playing through scenarios as to what might happen to the latter when its necessary population threshold is gone. Civilization here can be understood to mean two things: firstly, the *force of law* and secondly the formation of *civil society* in which relationality between subjects within the population is managed by both formal and informal frameworks of exchange, engagement, conviviality and governance. Foucault (2008: 295) viewed the concept of civil society as that field of reference through which governance technologies of power manage populations in ways distinct from, but interwoven with, the dominant neoliberal economic processes of markets, production, consumption and exchange. Civil society operates within an economic framework but for the purpose of ensuring that governmentality is not split between a branch of governing economically and a branch of governing juridically – that is, biopolitical governmentality operating within and on behalf of neoliberalism establishes civil society as a frame of reference. Civil society is the framework through which the workable bond of subjects is constituted.

For Foucault, civilizational governance emerges historically, in a modified form, from the pastoral care of the medieval church (Petterson 2012: 90–1) to produce disciplinary institutions and, later, biopolitical and security forms of governance that 'look after' groups and populations; in doing so, such post-pastoral governance technologies produce a spontaneous bond of individual subjects:

> [T]here is no explicit contract, no voluntary union, no renunciation of rights, and no delegation of natural rights to someone else; in short, there is no constitution of sovereignty by a sort of pact of subjection. In fact, if civil society actually carries out a synthesis, it will quite simply be through a summation of individual satisfactions within the social bond itself.
>
> (Foucault 2008: 300)

It operates, then, as the matrix of political and social power that permits neo-liberal economic technologies of power to flourish without dissent. At the same time, civil society provides a constitutive force for the social relationalities between subjects within a population grouping beyond the purely economic.

Apocalyptic film and television texts typically name civil society, civilization or society as that which is at risk, or that which has been lost in the course of the catastrophic spread of disease and the decimation of population. Civilization depends on population size that is not affected by a radical shift – only ever gradual, governed, managed growth or decline. In this respect, the disease is recognized as that which interrupts the management of the population size, resulting in the loss of shared social, biopolitical and juridical services (water, social security, health security, communications infrastructure, law, a legislative framework for criminal responsiveness and forms of policing) and economic fields of exchange (industrial production of food and agriculture, the supply of supermarkets, electricity, communications infrastructure), noting that many of these services are both economic and civil or shift between the two in recent Western history.

Where the West remains, very much problematically, the representation of progress and, as Stephen Muecke (2007: 260) has described, the depiction of 'man's sense of mastery of "nature"', what is lost in the loss of civilization is capability for survival – whether that be the infrastructure and knowledge frameworks that enable the mass growth and distribution of food, the taming of animals (dogs losing their companion species status and forming wild packs that compete with humanity being a common theme in apocalyptic texts) or the labour force capable of developing a vaccine or cure (noting that some of the 'happier ending' apocalyptic texts such as *Contagion* represent vaccine development, manufacture and distribution as the implausible work of a single, clever scientist working alone). Across these texts is the idea that civilization is, itself, precarious. Concepts of precarity, as Butler (2009: 13–14) points out, demand 'certain social and economic conditions to be met' in order to sustain life, and this includes specifically 'living socially' – that is, living amongst population that is not only a population of people but also a population in relationality arranged through obligations of civil society as the means of sustaining life.

The precarity of civilization depicted in apocalyptic media is very often one which operates at the connection between the *city* (as the figurative visual representation of civil society) and *global movement* (as the framework by which not only viruses travel but also the trade routes that underpin contemporary exchange). As Mark Poster (2001) has argued, the increasing globalization of economic processes has resulted in production and services being dispersed beyond the local, and these have occurred in ways which may produce increased profit (for some) but also increased inequity (for others) and substantial precarity (for all). Within an industrialized and mechanized society, any capacity to have agency over the forms of civility, the infrastructure for sustenance or the means of survival is lost as it is spread further through stratified systems, broad populations or globalized spaces. When the population that participates in (but does not govern) such services, goods and civil forms is gone, they themselves cannot be recuperated back to the individual who remains permanently alienated from them. The loss of such civil society that becomes at least one of the focal points for the disruption of identity in apocalyptic narratives, explicitly pointing to the contemporary reliance on these services that are not only for the flourishing of life, but also for the making of life *liveable* and the making of subjects intelligible in relationality to each other. In other words, a threshold of population is required for civil society to operate, and when that threshold is no longer met or radically disrupted, we see that there is no distinction between civil society and population whatsoever, and thus no subject that is not conditioned and constituted by population in radical and deep interdependency.

The shifts in identity, relationality and culture that occur in a movement away from civil society resulting from de-population are very neatly articulated in the 1984 nuclear apocalypse film *Threads*. The film's documentary-style voice-over begins with a statement that points to the relationship between contemporary civilization and a sustainably large population, in which society is depicted as, itself, susceptible at the point of that relationship:

> In an urban society, everything connects. Each person's needs are fed by the skills
> of many others. Our lives are woven together in a fabric. But the connections
> that make a society strong also make it vulnerable.

The vulnerability of contemporary civilization depicted in *Threads* is the lack of skills among survivors of an apocalyptic catastrophe resulting from their present global dispersal – that is, the skills for international trade of basic needs such as food, water, shelter, clothing and education.

The attachment to the urban-global connection becomes, in many such texts, an anxiety for the individual survivor and, thus, for the audience for whom they represent in prompting the recognition of individual vulnerability from a lack of capability to care for the self outside the radical interdependency of members of a population engaged in civil society. In the 1970s iteration of the television series *Survivor*, in which an influenza-like disease decimates the majority of people across the globe, key character Abby encounters a surviving schoolteacher while looking for her missing son. They have a conversation about food, education and manufacturing that helps shape her views of the future for the survivors, particularly after he explains the finite possibilities of scavenging existing food supplies:

> Schoolteacher: What is important is learning again. Things you've never even
> needed to consider before. [He points to a candle]. That: could you make that?
> Where does the raw material come from, do you know?… could you make it,
> something as simple as a candle, starting from scratch …. A book will tell you
> how electricity is generated, but could you do it?

That is, manufacturing, as a conceptual marker of civilization, has been dependent on quantum of people. In the 2008 version of the series, a similar situation arises, in which a more contemporary Abby – likewise searching for her son – encounters not a reflective, philosophical master but a physical education instructor. They have, however, a similar conversation with some marked differences after the instructor sees Abby once again trying her mobile phone:

> Brown: We're going to have to start all over again. We're going to have to re-learn the skills we've forgotten. We've become like helpless babies. Pushing the buttons of our fancy technology, while distancing ourselves further every day from the reality of what it actually is to *be* human.

While the 1970s iteration presents an apocalyptic scenario in which the reflection is the impossibility of recovery because to be human is to be *interdependent*, the 2008 depiction is more masculinist in arguing that the lost *individualized* survival skills is what constitutes human identity.

That which is vulnerable in apocalyptic depictions is therefore not population as a *large number* of human beings. Rather, it is the interdependent network of industrialized processes, relations, socialities and administrative governance forms that operate as a network. Contemporary society built on a particular countable number of people in a population who work together to produce a particular way of being is a network morphology, to use Manuel Castells' (2000) term, that structures relationality and identity in ways never free from structuration. That is, infrastructure and civilization sustain not just life but liveability, providing a framework for subjectivity that is produced in relation to one another. A subject comes to be a subject not by virtue of process of subjectification but in forms of network relationality that positions a subject within interdependency through nodes and hubs of infrastructure from those which sustain bodies (water, food distribution) to those which provide it with civilized belonging (education, participation). What makes these texts apocalyptic, then, is the finality of the loss of civilization or the very near insurmountability of deliberately attempting to bring about its restoration in a de-populated world. To envisage a post-civilization subsequent to an apocalyptic event that has decimated population numbers is no longer to imagine how one might re-build civilization (or build it differently, or restore the population) but, instead, to imagine the difficulty of re-building without the technologies that emerge from large population numbers as being insurmountable.

During the COVID lockdowns in 2020 and 2021 in many parts of the world, the capacity of infrastructure to enable survival was not, itself, destroyed although certainly the sense that it was threatened was felt by some, and in ways which were inequitable. For example, although there had been some panic-buying in the early weeks of the pandemic that mirrored the kinds witnessed in apocalyptic film and television series and was indicative of a fear the civil infrastructure that enabled the purchase of necessities might fail (McMillan and Papworth 2020), most people in major Western cities in stable democracies around the world found they were well-served with a civilized infrastructure, law, alternative practices of purchasing necessities (food deliveries, online shopping) and the continuation of the electricity and communication services. The discovery that any fears of civil society's precarity were not realized was not, of course, evenly experienced around the globe. In 2022, residents in Shanghai found their lockdown measures to control an outbreak resulted in the failure of health infrastructures and the delivery of food supplies (Kuo et al. 2022), presenting an alarming example of civilizational collapse in a sophisticated urban setting.

While civil society operates as a social framework, subjects are made vulnerable without an intelligible sense of 'civilization' and its role in structuring broad, social relationality. As Butler (2009: 25–6) points out, the state and the law can protect subjects, although to be protected by the state is to always be exposed to the violence wielded by the state, such that there is never any framework in which subjects are not already produced in vulnerability, only that vulnerability is produced and accorded differentially across different spaces and temporalities. Vulnerability, indeed, is a key condition of subjectivity. We experience vulnerability as corporeal beings who are dependent on others for physical support and survival from the very beginning of our lives. What we are vulnerable to is not merely the corporeal violences of hunger, disease or exposure. Rather, vulnerability is also always from the beginning about the possibility of loss, and this is where it is constitutive of our identities:

This means that each of us is constituted politically in part by virtue of the social vulnerability of our bodies – as a site of desire and physical vulnerability, as a site of a publicity at once assertive and exposed. Loss and vulnerability seem to follow from our being socially constituted bodies, attached to others, at risk of losing those attachments, exposed to others, at risk of violence by virtue of that exposure.

(Butler 2003: 20)

While we ordinarily perceive loss, grief and mourning in the context of those others whom we know and love, our more tacit but substantially important attachment to the civil society that provides (unevenly) the infrastructural supports for interdependency and mutual care is recognized as something that *can* be lost, thereby positioning us in a melancholic relationship in which we postpone mourning that loss by watching it play out in apocalyptic texts.

Melancholic attachments

By describing our cultural narratives of apocalyptic stories not as a roadmap for how to behave consciously in the context of a pandemic but as something which cues a deep-seated psychic response to the catastrophe of a pandemic, I am suggesting these narratives operate as a means of processing a melancholic attachment to the two figures of stable population and civil society, both of which are depicted in apocalyptic texts as precarious and capable of being lost. Butler (1997: 29), drawing on Freud, notes that while we grieve that which is lost as an ordinary process, in the case of that which has been or may be lost that is too harmful to our identities to confront, we face the situation of a melancholia that operates at the very limits of subjectivity. By transferring our concerns about the precarity of population (not individuals) and civilization (that enables liveability) into the realms of apocalyptic film and television rather than engaging with it critically as part of the practice of understanding the spatial and conceptual settings we cohabit as subjects, we disavow the actual precarities of both. Melancholia is always the failure to acknowledge the reality that something can be lost (Butler 2020: 166), thereby incorporating that loss (past or potential) into the self at the psychic level, always turned on the self in damaging ways.

This problematically leaves us with the inaccurate impression that the wider population will be 'fine', that mortality will not radically alter the make-up of the globe's inhabitants and the civil society founded in law, exchange, supply, trade, movement, labour and consumption will (and must) persist albeit with minor, unavoidable ripples. In other words, the cultural practice of consuming apocalyptic narratives in one setting enables the erroneous sense of society's inviolability, with repercussions for how we therefore think about disease. COVID-19 becomes, in this frame, a site of anxiety because it is perceived to affect the individual body, make the body sick, rather than be recognized as something threatening to the two elements of peopleness and civilization that enable contemporary, stable identity. At the same time, the melancholic attachment to these two sponsors some of the more inexplicable behaviours of COVID-deniers – not those who have cleverly monetized disinformation but those who take up and embrace the conspiratorial belief that there never was a virus. In this case, engaging with apocalyptic texts may provide the solution to providing the release that prevents melancholia overwhelming the self, although of course a critical engagement with how sociality is arranged would undoubtedly be better.

Conclusion

Human subjectivity is constituted in an attachment to diversely interpreted but shared concepts of civilization, stability and community or relationality. Given their significance in the very sense of selfhood, that attachment must be mourned in advance. Just as with an attachment to life, a cultural melancholia is established within the dual framework of the need to mourn that which will pain us if lost, and the need to put off that mourning in order to pursue liveable lives. In the case of the attachment to civilization, stable population, stability of population health, the shared production and distribution of goods that serve essential needs, mobility through space and infrastructures for living, mourning is both enacted and postponed through the cultural pleasures of popular apocalyptic film and television which regularly rank as the most popular fictional on-screen entertainment consumed in Anglophone countries.

One cultural purpose of the consumption of such texts is to sustain the attachment to the nexus between a living human population and a perception of civilization. it does so by creating the melancholic conditions of grievability of civilization's precarity by providing narratives of civilization's vulnerability that have the force of myth. At the same time, of course, such cultural narratives act as a 'lightening rod' that draws attention away from genuine precarity, such that these films and texts operate as a separate site for expressing and exploring that grievable precarity, allowing a sense of everydayness, stability and temporal sameness to persist.

One example of how the cultural narratives of precarity depicted in apocalyptic film and television texts inform COVID-19 responses includes the more extreme example of conspiracy theories related to government origins of the SARS-CoV-2 virus, conditioning members of the public who were previously uninitiated into conspiracy theory networks to find an explanatory discourse in the idea of a 'deep state' developing the virus for illicit purposes. While it is widely recognized of course that all genomic testing of the virus indicates there is no possibility it is artificial, laboratory-created or interfered with in any technological way (Anderson et al. 2020; Tellier 2020), the narrative that it is a laboratory-created weapon either for military use in conquest or for application by a secret government to control its own people draws on the discourses made available in apocalyptic film and television. That is, although conspiracy theories have been activated and sustained through the use of social networks supported by high-profile but outsider figures (Romer and Jamieson 2020) and the interrelationship of existing and new conspiracy theories (Miller 2020), the conditions that create a social logic for such outlandish ideas that a virus resulted from a hidden government agenda rather than encroachment into parts of the world ordinarily not traversed by human subjects is 'made available' through the discourses of apocalyptic film and television. To put this in cultural studies terms, apocalyptic film and television, the repetition of its narratives over time and the resultant wide recognizability of its discourses provide an opportunity not to consider what course of action we might take or how the pandemic might unfold, but a cultural mechanism to disavow consideration of several *realities*, whether the origins of the virus, the precarity of populations and civil structures or the very fact of our interdependency necessary for survival.

3

Disrupted identity: The self in a time of radical cultural change, anxiety and crisis

Introduction

Over the past chapters I have discussed three broad knowledge frameworks that guide public sphere discourse on the COVID-19 pandemic: the formation of cultural rupture in storytelling of crisis and resilience, the set of competing media frameworks that establish a complex matrix of information across which one must plot one's identity, behaviour and belonging, and the role of apocalyptic storytelling that cues particular responses to disease in ways which establish anxieties over the security of civilization itself. In this chapter, I would like to turn now to how we can theorize precisely how identity is re-formed and re-constituted in the context of the kinds of substantial disruption to normative, everyday liveability that the pandemic and its protective measures brought, and what this means for the how we understand selfhood in terms of sociality, relationality and belonging.

The most sophisticated humanities approach to identity is Butler's (1990, 1993) theory of identity performativity which draws on both poststructuralist and psychoanalytic concepts to argue that self-identity is not an innate, essentialist inner core that drives particular actions and behaviours, but is constituted precisely in our non-voluntarist, unconscious performances of selfhood. Such performances, articulations, attitudes and ways-of-being are governed by norms given in language, culture and discourse (including media) in ways that discipline us into practices that help us fulfil the cultural demand for intelligibility, coherence and recognizability in order to participate socially and belong. Stabilizing over time, the performances of our self-identity and the formations of identity that operate alongside axes of discrimination (gender, race, ethnicity, physical ability) and other distinctions call upon us to practice identities in ways which lend the illusion that there is an individual, core self with agency.

An argument here, however, is that such an illusion is based on the production and performance of the self in a coherent, linear pattern over time, and that depends on certain stabilities across the everydayness of daily life. As subjects and as human beings, we cohere our liveability and performativity through cyclical patterns across days, weeks and years. Movement in and out of the home, movement to and from places of work, shopping, social engagement, kinship visits and health practitioners, from residence to places of holiday and exploration, and from through patterns of movement of residences and changing homes are among components that *mark* those patterns of everydayness. Of course, this capacity to enjoy stable patterns of everydayness and movement is not equally or democratically available to all, but our perception of these as a dominant and colonizing Western norm is significant in the intelligibility and recognizability of our identities to ourselves and others. We need to ask, then, what happens when these are disrupted: the inability to move from places of sleep to places of work, to participate in daily cycles of attendance at a gym or social venue, to engage in the mundane activities of grocery shopping, to plan holidays and escapes, to perceive a future (next day or next year) grounded in the linear normativity that enables stable performativities?

To address the ways in which the pandemic can be understood as a disruption of the conditions that enable a linear performativity of identity, I will begin with a brief summary of the key tenets in understanding identity as performative and constituted in discourses of the everyday before considering how 'ruptured time' shifts the grounds by which identity is made intelligible. I would then like to address the corporeal aspects of identity to show that what was revealed in acts of hoarding food, toilet paper and other goods normally associated with the base conditions of bodily liveability is a deep-seated anxiety over identity. I will then make some remarks on the ways in which interdependency is a significant spectral aspect of coherent identity and how a perception of disrupted futurity interrupts that coherence.

Identity performativity and cultural normativity

If identity is performed in accord with discourse, relationality and cultural norms, then the disruption to these three elements of everyday life that was caused by the onset of the pandemic as 'crisis' and the sustained health measures establishes a situation in which the intelligibility and coherence of identity is itself disrupted. We can make sense of this in considering Butler's framework of the performativity of identity and its capacity to be reconstituted in the 'encounter' with the rupture and the emergence of the new. Working from a post-structuralist and anti-foundationalist perspective that draws on Foucault, Lacan and Derrida, Butler's theory of performativity is based on the idea that identity and subjectivity is an ongoing *process* of becoming, rather than an ontological state of being, whereby *becoming* is a sequence of acts that retroactively constitutes identity (Butler 1990). That is, the performance of a facet of identity draws on the demands of a discursively given knowledge framework that establishes the necessary fiction of an actor behind the act, a doer behind the deed. The self or 'I' is made up of a matrix of identity categories, experiences and labels (Butler 1990: 40) that, through repetition sustained over time, lend the *illusion* of an inner identity core driving those actions (Butler 1993: 12). Although Butler's work is complex and wide-ranging, there are three core nodes of her approach to identity performativity which are significant for understanding how identity stability is achieved through reiterative performativity, the citation of discourses and everyday cultural practices.

Firstly, building on the work of earlier theorists such as Nietzsche, Foucault and Lacan, Butler (1990) argued that there is no knowable core essence or inner self from which behaviours and actions emerge, nor an inner agency that drives voluntary decisions over identity, self-presentation and subjectivity. Rather, there are only sets of performances that retroactively produce an illusion of an inner identity core. That is, there is no doer behind the deed, no actor behind the acts. The sense we have of an inner identity self is only ever an *effect* of those performances (Butler 1993: 12). In this respect, our identities are shaped by the available practices, actions and behaviours that enable coherence and intelligibility as selves by coming to seem and feel 'natural' and 'everyday', hidden from conscious reflection. When everydayness and the spatial, corporeal and relational aspects are suddenly shifted – as they were in the onset of the pandemic and the health measures taken to prevent the spread of the virus, the terrain through which our performances of selfhood are made was substantially disrupted, re-framing that which makes such performances intelligible to ourselves.

Secondly, our identities are performed 'in accord' with discursively given norms, categories, stereotypes, labels and expressions. These norms are given to us in culture, and while we vary them substantially an aspect of that normativity is their persistence over time. We see this, for example, in the deployment of stereotypes governing particular identity behaviours that continue over time despite critique (Rosello 1998). Norms given in discourse and culture are not, of course, as constraining as stereotypes or closely disciplined behaviours. Rather, as we know from Foucault (2008: 259–60), they vary and fluctuate in order not to be contested. However, there are limits to the extent to which the norm is permitted to vary, what Foucault (2007: 63) identified as distributional 'curves of normality' that allow diversity within a range. When those regulatory norms (Butler 1990: 32) are not in the control of the disciplinary and biopolitical institutions that reinforce and repeat such curves of normality, such as when an unexpected, unanticipated pandemic disrupts the practice of repetition of those norms (e.g. labourers of particular types attend their workplaces on a Monday morning), then the limits of those curves are tested, calling upon people to plot themselves *beyond* the bounds of normativity. Here, again, the cultural grounding by which identities are reproduced through intelligibility (e.g. that the labourer who fails to attend work without good reason is marked as unintelligible – not recognized as a subject) then we once again find the possibilities of coherent identity put in question.

Finally, the process of performing identity within regimentary norms occurs within a narrative of coherence *over time*, motivated by a cultural demand or imperative that we are coherent, intelligible and recognizable to others in order to allow social participation and belonging (Butler 1997: 27). That includes intelligibility to the self as well as to others in order to take part in relationality and social life. When the two aspects of identity disruption described above take place, the capacity to be an intelligible subject to oneself and others *over time* is also disrupted, calling upon the subject to reflect on one's own performativity. Here is where one of Butler's key arguments about repetition is at play – our identities are coherent over time because we insistently repeat them in order to be coherent. However, when the capacity to repeat is damaged by sudden, changing social relations, we are positioned to ask ourselves *how* to repeat in order to remain intelligible. Genuine repetition is, of course, mythical since the conditions that make an exact repetition of a prior moment have changed in the very fact that moment cannot come again. Rather, repetition *must* conceal itself and the discontinuities that always are part of the inherent failure to repeat seamlessly (Butler 1990: 135–6), or else the very grounding of intelligible identities 'will be displaced and revealed as a stylized configuration, indeed, a … corporealization of time' (Butler 1990: 140–1). In the disruption of the order to, say, stay at home, to change one's 'natural' behaviour, to cease repeating the norms that make us stable identities, the ground by which identity is made intelligible over time is revealed, displacing its hiddenness and stability, and calling upon us to re-figure or re-constitute as something other.

Certainly, part of the 'shock' of the onset of the pandemic and the disruption to everyday life can be read not merely through lenses of fear, anxiety, risk, apprehension over the continuity of health, well-being, economies or social lives (although of course these remain a part of the picture). Rather, the 'shock' of the crisis and rupture to everyday cultural norms is a crisis for selfhood itself. For some, the disruption of normative identity regimes was expressed in anger, outrage or panic. For some, relationships broke down. For many, a reflection on what *kind* of identity one had, such as an identity foregrounded on particular jobs, resulted in decisions to break with that identity and choose alternative work or no work – what has been called the 'Great Resignation' (Knott 2021a). Others chose to break with identities based on urban living to re-imagine a subjectivity in rural areas and a slower pace of life – what has been described for some as 'an unexpected opportunity to escape the rat race' (Fitzsimmons and Snow 2020). Although changes to work routines, concerns about illness, the reduction in noise from urban environments put into relative stillness all contribute to reflection on what it means to live and *how* to live a liveable life, the disruption of identity, subjectivity and selfhood – that we can apprehend if we think it in terms of performativity – in this unprecedented way calls upon us to meet the broader cultural demands of intelligibility be being re-constituted anew.

Constituting the self in ruptured time

It might be said that one aspect of middle-class, Western existence is the ironic desire for both consistency and novelty. We experience consistency in our engagement with the everyday – homes with which we are familiar arranged in ways that are not persistently changing; work routines that vary but not too much; computer interfaces and social media platforms that allow habitual engagement and are at least a little annoying when they change without notice; familiar friends, family and relationships, and the people who must be rejected from those flows of affection when they change too quickly or in ways which are not recognizable and intelligible to us. At the same, there is a desire for novelty, variation and distraction that sits alongside consistency and familiarity, whether in the sexual desires of people who are otherwise attached by practices of monogamy (Schofield 1976: 134), the desire for television programming and streaming that entertains by providing the right mix of the familiar and the novel (Silverstone 1981: 82) or the limited-time escape from everydayness through holidays, travel and tourism (Urry 2007).

Such an embrace of the novel is part of what Pat Califia (1994: 151) identified as 'the human need for adventure, risk, competition, self-display, pleasurable stimulation, and novelty'. Yet it is always limited by nature. For John Caputo (1993), novelty is a core aspect of ethical practices of identity in relation to belonging to communities. An ethical community calls for being bound to the good of the community without sacrificing diversity (273n50), and that diversity is enabled not by a postmodern individualism or collapse into singularity but through the practice and embrace of novelty, understood as 'new ways to be (*renovatio*), putting on a new life, in indefinitely many ways' (41). Another way to perceive this is that the limits on novelty serve to reinforce and *make apparent* the familiar – change that is incremental and manageable through a sense of agency is acceptable, but that which is not is *disruption*. Many people (myself included) undoubtedly found the early days of the pandemic and the necessary health restrictions an exciting novelty, despite the concern and apprehension that the unfamiliarity of changed routines, mobility restrictions and unknowability brought. However, the more that novelty edged towards zones of non-agentic unknowability, the less that novelty confirmed the familiar and the more *liminal* it became.

Liminality, defined as the quality of ambiguity of being located physically, emotionally, culturally or in terms of identity in a space or time of threshold (Turner 1969), is a useful way of framing the contemporary situation of COVID-19, particularly in terms of the temporality involved in anticipating one of the newly available vaccines might restore normality. Or in the terms of a virus the longer-term effects on otherwise healthy bodies of which is as yet not fully known and, of course, in terms of the length of lockdown and social distancing measures, or the consistency of employment, or bans on international travel, among many other examples of unknowable time. The long period before coming through anything that resembled the familiarity of the normal everyday, the more the pandemic must therefore be defined as a cultural rupture to the *temporal* frames by which identity is made intelligible.

What, then, does that rupture do for identity recognized as performative? Butler's framework of making sense of the performativity of the subject is all very well in the *ordinary* course of history, culture and discourse represented through the pivots of the familiar and the novel but always perceived and apprehended as stable or, through reflection, as slow-changing. When discourse, culture, history and the everyday familiar are radically disrupted by a pandemic that encourages panic, economic and political restructuring, states of exception, restrictions on everyday mobility, significant changes for many in the routines of labour and consumption, sudden unemployment, sudden unavailability of the ordinary practices of social engagement and other aspects upon which the bourgeois normative figure is constituted as an intelligible and recognizable subject, we are called upon not merely to accept the destabilization of identity but to re-constitute ourselves in difference.

An aspect of performative identity that stems from Butler's work which is less-often invoked is that of transformation or re-constitution. The obscurity of this concern is most likely the result of the preoccupation with the ways in which we come to perform fictionally 'fixed' identity categories, rather than how they are diverted, morphed, transmuted. Butler provides a useful example related to sexual identity: concerning how the category of selfhood represented by the 'I' comes to perform a lesbian identity that stabilizes partially through repetitive citation, she suggests that: 'It is through the repeated play of this sexuality that the "I" is insistently reconstituted as a lesbian "I"; paradoxically it is precisely the *repetition* of that play that establishes as well the *instability* of the very category that it constitutes' (Butler 1991: 18). Underlying this notion of reconstitution is what is perhaps best referred to as an *encounter*: the 'I' can be reconstituted as a different kind of 'I' through the repeated play and performance of the category and its recognizable, intelligible codes of behaviour and desire, but *only* within the context of having encountered new discourses, relationalities and normative frames of cultural practice that were not previously available and that establish a new logic of selfhood.

Although Butler was discussing reconstitution in terms of sexual subjectivity – which is perhaps to be seen as more malleable since sexuality and sexual orientation fixates on something which is 'inaugurated' at a particular point on the threshold between the different discourses of childhood and young adulthood (Cover 2019) – the conceptualization of identity *change* provides a way of making sense of what happens to identity when we perceive the pandemic as a temporal rupture between the past norms of everyday familiarity and the cultural contingencies, practices, restrictions and anxieties over the crisis of the pandemic. That is, in the encounter with the changed circumstances of the world, mobility, time, space, relationships and consumption brought about by

COVID-19, the sudden re-framing of public sphere discourse in the biopolitical language of population health, the persistent deployment of new disciplinary measures designed to protect or enhance subjects in changed circumstances, the apocalyptic rhetoric operating in some sectors, the contestation and uncertainty of protest in some cities, the subject is insistently re-constituted in the loss of the constitutive discursive and cultural force of the *prior* everyday, and transformed through the encounter with liminality, unknowability and new chrononormativities.

For Butler (1990: 15), *transformation* of the subject is possible only through a rejection of any identity foundation, which she sees as foreclosing in advance the 'emergence of new identity concepts' and the 'transformation or expansion of existing identity concepts'. Such transformative potential as given in poststructuralist accounts is neither a complete rejection of identity as a cultural process, nor a suggestion that fragmentary and contradictory identities are possible outside of a cultural concept of internal unity (Connolly 1991: 178). Rather, the transformation of the self into new identity configurations occurs in the practice of encountering that which produces not only changes in self-definition but also bodily effects (Cooper 2000: 108). The affective sense of disruption or transformation of the self, juxtaposed with the cultural demands for self-consistency and unity, establishes an *identity anxiety* that is both bodily and relational, discharging the subject of subjectivity and insisting that subjects find new groundings for coherent performativity of the self.

What is experienced in the COVID-19 disruption to subjectivity is a liminal passage towards that as-yet unknowable altered subjecthood. The loss of *coherent* subjectivity that is produced by the cultural rupture of drastic and sudden change to the everyday requires grieving. Like all identity loss, change or disruption there is a practice of *mourning* that must be undergone before transformation and re-constitution can take place. In the context of COVID-19, we see grieving not for those who have been infected or died of the illness, but grieving expressed through anger, outrage and rejection of the requirements for social distancing and immobility. Such practices of grieving for the lost prior self in the era of COVID-19 are best witnessed, perhaps, in the protests in the United States against the health protection and bio-safety measures put in place in several states: examples include attempts to find a discursive grounding for the unknowable by harking back to lost intelligibilities through disavowal of the reality of the pandemic, by looking for coherence in drawing together a conspiracy theory narrative about 5G mobile telecommunications, by focusing protest about the pandemic measures through issues related anti-Biden dissent, pro-Trump rallying and outrage over more restrictive gun ownership laws and – of course – anti-vaccination rhetoric. This assembling of bodies to protest is in the form identified by Butler (2015: 9) that galvanizes around certain claims to vulnerability. While much protest over vulnerability relates to the inequitable distribution of precarity, in this case, the protests, outrage, disavowal and denial might better be seen as a response to the kinds of vulnerabilities of identity that occur in the context of being called upon to re-constitute oneself as a subject in ruptured and radically changed cultural circumstances. In that sense, for those un-resourced to re-constitute a sense of identity and liveability, such outrage, disavowal and protest can be seen as a fruitless attempt to re-assert a sense of identity *dignity* which, as Francis Fukuyama (2019) has argued, is central to the practice of twenty-first-century subjectivity. Dignity here emerges as denial of the revelation of identity's inherent instability and the way it shows up in the context of cultural rupture.

Anxiety, bodies and subjectivity

Having addressed how some of the ways in which the loss of identity due to the sudden rupture of cultural normativities have come into play, it is valuable to turn to some of the ways in which we can understand identity disruption in terms of corporeality and the embodied framework through which performativity is mechanized. A notable experience in the early months of the COVID-19 crisis in many Western countries was the unexpected – and often illogical – panic-buying and hoarding of toilet paper (Fisher 2020, Mao 2020, Moore 2020). Rather than the staples of panic-buying and hoarding more recognizable in the apocalyptic screen media discussed in the previous chapter such as food, cash, petrol, batteries or books, toilet paper was (literally) fought over in supermarkets by people filling trolleys of a supply that would last years. The fact that it is this bodily function to which attention turned was surprising (especially given the uninterrupted capability to wash rather than wipe). However, when we consider how this particular panic emerges in the context of a re-constitution of selfhood it begins to make more sense.

I would like to make the case here that the concentration on toilet paper rather than other more urgent aspects of survival such as food is indicative not of a panicked response to the declaration of emergency and pandemic, but a symptom of the reconstitutive formation of the crisis and rupture which creates a disturbance in selfhood not as a psychic being but at the very level of subjective corporeality. This disturbance should not be read as the change in subjectivity itself, but as the liminal passage through which a focus on very basic bodily needs becomes the site of attachment and worry while new configurations of identity intelligibility, normativity and selfhood stabilize (Cover 2013a: 417). The disturbance here is, indeed, very specifically one which draws attention to the body as an object of fixation through which subjectivity attempts to stabilize itself in the process of transformation. The self lived as a corporeal subject is, of course, markedly significant for the understanding of vulnerability and the precarity of life whereby the risk of illness or accident is 'built into the very conception of bodily life ... always given over to modes of sociality and environment that limit its individual autonomy' (Butler 2009: 30–1). The subject's vulnerability is highlighted (to oneself and to each other) by the very basic *bodily needs* that draw attention to the precarity of subjecthood: toilet and hygiene. Indeed, this serves as an explanatory framework for the radical hoarding of – and obsessive discourse upon – toilet paper at the beginning of the COVID-19 crisis, and in many subsequent experiences of temporary lockdown, particularly in Australia, the United States and the UK.

The re-constitution of the performative self in the context of the cultural rupture brought about by COVID-19 and its changes to everyday mobility is thus something which prompted a re-configuration of subjectivity in such a dramatic way as to give focus on the most base aspect of the body: its excretion. As a disturbance in selfhood, or what Cathy Caruth (1995: 154) refers to as an 'event's essential incomprehensibility', the force of its *affront to understanding*, the performance of the subject vis-à-vis relationality with the other and with space and time is radically re-oriented – the logic through which the normal, temporal activities of the body such as excretion are so radically made to feel precarious that people were willing to fight each other to buy toilet paper. It is tempting, of course, to consider a psychoanalytic framework here, although once we are thinking about the reconstitutive force of the cultural rupture we can see instead that it is not within the context of a disrupted psyche that people turned their attention to the most base of bodily functions, but through the disturbance to the 'I'; a re-constituted subjectivity that recognizes the simultaneous vulnerability of the self and the precarity of ways-of-being that we ordinarily frame as civilization (Cover 2013a). One is not re-constituted as a subject fixated on basic bodily functions; rather, the sudden attachment to an anxiety over the body's base functions is an *effect* of the process of identity transformation, re-constitution and re-stabilization through which such anxieties naturally dissipate.

The toilet paper example is, of course, the most severe expression of the kind of anxiety produced in the reconstitution of subjectivity produced by the sudden cultural affront of COVID-19. Alongside the disavowal of COVID-19's reality, the protests and the more common baffled silence and resigned compliance of the majority, it is a useful reminder that while the effects of the response to COVID-19 can be rationalized, the very threat of the virus itself is a bodily one. Together with the destabilization of subjectivity caused by cultural rupture and sudden change and the demands for re-constitution of identity in the encounter with discourses and everyday practices that had changed, the threat of the virus reminds us of the inherent vulnerability as subjects. Vulnerability is, ultimately, always about the body (Gilson 2011: 35), but it is in the context of cultural rupture that the unified coherence of the psychic mapping of selfhood and corporeal life is disturbed, re-configured and awaiting transformation into that which can be provided by the eventual stabilization of a new environment, culture, discourse, practice of relationality, capacity to figure oneself in terms of new movements and new stillnesses, and in the sense of chrononormative futurity.

Identity in competing concepts of interdependency

In the Introduction to this book, I made some remarks about the different ways in which resilience has been perceived, including a social ecology approach in which everyday people draw on peer networks, families, social supports, infrastructure, stable environments and other aspects of social connectedness as sources of resilience in order to 'bounce back' from adverse experiences. I argued there that this was one instance in which we see *interdependency* at play. Another is in terms of the two elements I have described in the previous chapter as part of what is lost or mourned through the cultural ritual of engaging with apocalyptic texts: radical depopulation and loss of civilization that depend on an interdependent population for its sustainability. Here, we might argue that identity in the face of COVID-19 is also re-constituted resulting from *changes* to our perception of interdependency.

Although I deal in the next chapter with questions about mobility, social isolation, lockdowns and how interdependency is both re-figured and sustained in contexts of immobility, it is notable here that interdependency as part of everydayness is experienced – albeit tacitly – through the familiarity of ordinary practices that generally depend on movement and mobility: shopping, work and social engagement. Here, the fact that we are thrown into relationality with others and interdependency on the social is invisibilized. As we engage in the world in the context of our identity coherence, the liberal-humanist myth of individualism, the mythical goal of independence and self-reliance and a sense of self-agency, we obscure the foundational interdependency of life by perceiving our bodily boundaries as individual ends rather than thresholds of interrelationality (Butler 2020: 16), abstracting ourselves from the perception of being social creatures *despite* the fact that we are doing the things that are precisely social within the *a priori* fact of being interdependent with others.

In three other respects, however, our social interdependency became more foregrounded in everyday lives through the change in practices which highlighted what is 'merely' a backdrop to everyday familiarity as the setting and condition for intelligible performativity of identity. One of these is the fact that a virus only transfers from body to body as a direct result of that interdependency through which we move through life in settings that involve contact with others. The anxieties, then, that were established as people radically distanced themselves – by choice or by mandate – from face-to-face sociality is an anxiety over how to navigate subjectivity when it is constituted in relationality first and *before* any sense or reliance on the myth of independence and individualism.

A second, however, was the extent to which the change in everyday practices and the adoption of less-familiar means of bringing in food through grocery deliveries to the home rather than shopping in person, meals through food delivery services relying on 'gig economy' labour (Bennett and Backholer 2021) and accessing other goods (through a very substantial increase in the delivery of packages to private homes) (Buhler 2020). As we know from Sarah Sharma's (2014) work, interdependency on others who perform deliveries, clear waste and prepare services for others is often obscured by occurring at night-time as part of a temporal order of inequality. The fact that such services became apparent as part of the radical shift in everyday practices is one which calls upon us to rethink our sense of individual autonomy and to recognize – in ways different from our ordinary, familiar performativity of identity – that we are constituted in relationality that relies on others rather than in a false sense of self-autonomy.

The third of these is communication infrastructures enabling connectivity and communication. The shift to video-conferencing as a major element in work practices and social life, the struggle with infrastructure that sometimes failed, the reliance on those with whom we share spaces to be silent in the background while we conducted an online meeting, the calls to workplace technicians or grandchildren to help fix digital communication problems – all of these highlight the dependence on others to enable at-distance communication as part of being social, communicative subjects. At the same time, telehealth appointments with medical practitioners rather than visits to a clinic or surgery highlighted for many the interdependency with a *range* of health practitioners and the complexities of navigating the means of sustaining health that, likewise, are often obscured in a simple general practitioner's appointment (Clun 2020). Here, the *fact* of being interdependent subjects through communication became a key talking point of how we navigated the pandemic and, more pertinently, how we navigated the re-configured setting in which we practice and perform identity.

In all three of these cases, our interdependency, our thrownness into and reliance on sociality to connect, to eat and to communicate becomes foregrounded in everyday life. The shift of that interdependency from being a background experience to one that is obvious in the uncertainty of its continuation and availability is re-constitutive of identity. When our identities are constituted in a discourse that *pretends* self-reliance, individualism and independence not only as a liberal-humanist ideal but also as the practice on which coherence and intelligibility as individualized subjects is dependent (Butler 2020: 37–8), the radical foregrounding of that interdependency of our social existences likewise calls for a re-configuration of identity. As Sharma (2014: 12) notes, making the distinctions that obscure our interdependency and reliance on others who perform labour in obscured ways can be considered 'ruptural performances as part of [a] temporal insurgency'. We might read that in reverse: the temporal rupture of the pandemic and its health measures is one which re-figures performances based on *not knowing* just how interdependent we are. No longer are we able to presume ourselves as individuals bound together by a liberal social contract, but are required to acknowledge that interdependency in new ways. While there was, of course, a reasonable hope among many that this foregrounding might result in new ethical relations (Faine 2021), a return of pre-neoliberal state welfare (Jackson 2020), and other changes to our social, working and consumption practices, the change that was experienced for many was one in the very constitution of subjectivity that was re-figured through a heightened relationality and interdependency.

Conclusion

I have argued in this chapter that the COVID-19 pandemic and the health responses and mandates designed to prevent its spread were not only a disruption of everyday life, but that this disruption created the conditions for a radical shift in identity. If identity is understood as performative and therefore reliant on the consistency and 'slow change' of discourse, culture, practice and sociality, then a sudden shift removes the foundational cultural, temporal and linguistic environment in which identity is constituted. Where we are constituted in a mix of familiarity and a desire for novelty, change is acceptable and is, itself, familiar. However, when that novelty becomes radical disruption or rupture of the everyday in ways that are outside agency and control, we are called upon to re-constitute ourselves in a process of becoming that involves becoming something other. Identity does not dissolve, given the significance of the deeper cultural demand for coherence, intelligibility and recognizability in order to maintain social participation and belonging. Rather, it destabilizes calling upon us to re-stabilize ourselves.

Part of that instability is, I have argued, experienced through an over-determined attachment to the corporeal whereby the panic-buying and hoarding of toilet paper (of all things) can be understood as an *effect* of identity instability rather than a rational choice about what is needed to get through a lockdown. At the same time, the heightened recognition of the interdependency of human life to survive that was brought by the shift in practices of health, consumption and communication always warrants a re-constitution in undoing the mythical force of individualism, self-reliance and autonomy. It is too soon, of course, to apprehend whether these changes produce a more ethical way of being and performing liveability, but it is certainly possible to argue that the shifts in identity practices are likely to be as long-lasting as the health, economic and social impacts of the virus itself.

4

Disrupted mobility: Lockdowns, borders and movement

Introduction

In some respects, the performativity of identity is enabled by *mobility* and *movement* among the wider range of 'articulations' of the self (speech, deportment, actions). That is, if identity is articulated in repetitive ways that stabilize the illusion of an inner identity core (Butler 1990), and if identity is always relational and performed in the context of an interdependent social existence played out in space, then how we move about the world, how we embrace and breach the norms of mobility, how we engage socially through acts of normative economic activity, consumption, entertainment, labour, cultural relations, political processes and so on, are all expressions of identity. In other words, if an aspect of performativity involves movement and mobility, identity is the *effect* of such mobility, and movement through the world constitutes our sense of self and subjectivity.

What happens, then, to our practices and performances of identity when subjects are ordered into immobility, or when individuals are compelled to choose immobility and isolation for the safety of their own health? Immobility and stay-at-home orders have been a key health measure globally to prevent the spread of SARS-CoV-2 and its variants, to reduce the rate of transmission so as to alleviate over-burdened hospitals and medical professionals, and to provide time for the production and distribution of vaccines and anti-viral treatments. In different jurisdictions, immobility has taken the form of compulsory quarantine for those infected with the virus and/or those potentially exposed to infected persons, mandatory periods of quarantine for travellers coming into various countries, extended stay-at-home orders, 'work from home' requirements for those whose work allows, limitations on rights to cross borders and other lines demarcating movement restriction and in many regions limitations on the number of kilometres a person can travel from their ordinary place of residence.

I spent the first two years of the pandemic in Melbourne, Australia, which purportedly experienced one of the world's longest periods of lockdown by both consecutive and cumulative days across several separate mandatory stay-at-home orders (RMIT ABC Fact Check 2021). Melbourne experienced six periods of compulsory isolation and stay-at-home orders: an early lockdown of 43 calendar days in the first half of 2020; a second period of 111 consecutive days in the second half of 2020; three shorter lockdowns of 5, 14 and 12 days in the first half of 2021; and a final period of 77 calendar days in the second half of 2021 – a total of 262 days, which is a little over one-third of the days across two years, with other limitations on distance, movement between city and country.

At one level, this was an experience of relative isolation (self and partner) and a minor adjustment to having two people working daily at home. At a second level, it was a period of intense social and workplace engagement, in which I spent perhaps more time talking with others in what seemed like endless video-conference meetings with colleagues all over the globe. And at a completely different level, there was something at play that was, precisely, *not isolation* but the *shared experience* of living in a city of five million, most of whom were experiencing the same disruption of mobility restrictions (albeit in markedly different, often inequitable ways). Navigating these competing levels of experiencing something altogether new – restricted mobility – is not, I argue, a matter merely of mental health, resilience, getting on, coping or staying safe. Rather, it is a matter of mapping a substantial shift in spatial experience that impinges expressly on identity.

To make sense of the relationship between identity and the kinds of immobilities made necessary by protective health measures to stop the spread of serious virus, I will begin with a summary of some of the ways in which lockdowns and border closures has operated as a population health response, and how the cultural response to these was framed. I will then turn to how mobility can be apprehended as a matter of identity performativity, and the way in which mobility mechanizes social interdependency before a discussion of lockdowns as a perceived disturbance of subjectivity. I would like to end with a few remarks on how lockdowns have sometimes been discussed as a setting of isolation causing poor mental health, arguing that this limits a perspective on seeing the shared experience as a setting of social belonging.

Lockdowns as the form of immobility in COVID

Lockdowns, stay-at-home orders, mandatory isolation, quarantines and restrictions on border-crossing are all recognized mechanisms for the prevention of the spread of serious, communicable disease, and can be described as cultural and regulatory formations that prevent or reduce mobility and movement. They were deployed from early on in the pandemic as a key platform in the health and safety measures adopted by governments across much of the world – a substantial disruption to everyday life, work, leisure and travel, a shift in our perceived 'freedom' to move about within borders and without curfew and, as I argue below, a necessary adjustment to identity, subjectivity and belonging. Such measures were grounded in a perception of the social good – reducing the spread of the virus and therefore the relatively high mortality it wrought, alleviating hospitals and medical professionals, and buying the necessary time for the production of a vaccine.

The link between disease and mobility has long been recognized, dating back to ancient empires founded on movement, cities as gathering places, trade and military deployment, whereby a symbiotic link between the movement of people and disease was obvious and apparent (McNeill 1976: 126). The practice of restricting the movement of peoples (or animals) to prevent the spread of disease was not, of course, new. Some interpretation of passages in the Judeo-Christian Bible suggest that forms of quarantine were outlined in the requirement for those with leprosy to 'dwell apart' (Grisar 2020), although the form that quarantine, social isolation and restricted mobility takes today as a health measure has its origins in Mediaeval Europe. The term 'quarantine' itself is derived from the Venetian *quarantena* referring to the standard forty days of isolation of ships and visitors to prevent the spread of the Black Death (plague) during the mid-fourteenth century. As Foucault (2004b: 44–5) has pointed out, in the decades leading up to the early Enlightenment era, a practice of immobility founded on exclusion of the unwell began to be replaced by a more 'inclusive' practice of marking out territory and partitioning space to prevent the movement of the infected from an area of disease into an area free of disease.

The recognition of the connection between travel, movement and the spread of parasitic diseases such as bacterial infections and virus transmissions endures along an historical continuum to a contemporary recognition of the role of air travel in accelerating the diffusion of disease, but also homogenizing illness in ways which sometimes protect populations on a global scale (McNeill 1976: 14–15). Nevertheless, intervention in mobility has been the most obvious weapon against disease, whether that is not visiting one's grandparents while having a cold to isolating hospital patients with Staphylococcal infections from other, uninfected patients. In other words, the concept of 'spread' and the cultural formation of 'mobility' are entangled, such that the mediaeval recognition of the movement of rats and the contemporary understanding that an overseas trip risks 'catching' a cold is deeply ingrained in cultural health practices. In that respect, anyone who is aware of those histories would not be at all surprised that the immediate response of governments – whether operating through the sovereignty of the interventional executive order (Lemke 2011: 98–9) or the biopolitical regime of tracking communicable disease through global health surveillance (Ostherr 2004: 300) – was immediately put in the position of having to restrain mobility as the principal means by which a virus is transmitted despite the fact, as I argue below, mobility is *also* the principal means by which subjectivity is performed as an interrelational being thrown into sociality.

Indeed, for Foucault, aspects of the nineteenth- and twentieth-century forms of institutional and administrative discipline, surveillance and regulation of norms have their origins in the development of techniques that restrict mobility and movement as a response to plague in the early 1700s:

> These plague regulations involve literally imposing a partitioning grid on the regions and towns struck by plague, with regulations indicating when people can go out, how, at what times, what they must do at home, what type of food they must have, prohibiting certain types of contact, requiring them to present themselves to inspectors, and to open their homes to inspectors. We can say that this is a disciplinary type of system.
>
> (Foucault 2007: 10–11)

Here, disease, illness and infection become subject to an intersection between the *spatiality* of a town or city, and the bodies that the disciplinary measures seek to make normal and free from disease.

What has arguably been a tried-and-tested practice to prevent the spread of infection was the model, with some modification and variance, deployed around the world. However, for most people in Western regions, the 'idea' of quarantine is not something experienced through the demarcation of space (home/public, the establishment of new borders and checkpoints, the division of towns and cities within jurisdictions normally permitting free travel). Here, again, we have a framework of disruption that calls upon subjects to not only calculate a response, but where that response itself is a sustained set of performative acts that inculcates forms of subjectivity. So how can we describe the practice of response? Throughout much of the world where lockdown, stay-at-home, isolation and quarantine measures were deployed there was, of course, substantial compliance with these immobility practices – whether through fear or concern about catching COVID-19, broad agreement with the ethical reasons for not providing avenues for a killer virus to spread or general acquiescence to government regulatory measures and mandatory rules. However, there were two other kinds of response, both of which speak to the ways in which responding to restrictions on mobility operate within the competing discourses of subjectivity and identity in contexts of belonging.

The first and most 'visible' other kind of response was that of refusal and protest. Although occurring notably in the United States across jurisdictions that enforced lockdowns, many other countries also experienced protests – sometimes violent – over quarantine and stay-at-home regulations (Breakey 2021). Much of the protest movement that formed across the pre-vaccination years of the COVID-19 pandemic was based in a liberal-humanist and über-individualist set of beliefs that governments do not have a 'right' to restrict movement and mobility. This is a liberal assertion of identity in an Enlightenment context that presupposes the subject as a self-governing, natural person, able to make rational choices, act upon them and thereby 'influence intentionally the way the world goes' (Benn 1982: 4–5). Liberal philosopher John Locke attributed natural rights to this subject as a free and equal individual capable of consent to be governed (Locke 1988: 337–8, 428). For such protesters, the concept of the self-contained, self-present individual subject is supreme, with a natural right to 'liberty' – read and understood as a right to mobility and movement even during times of risk – and in which interference with such liberty is read as a form of totalitarian governance. Even in brands of liberalism that drew more obviously on John Stuart Mill's (1972) utilitarianism, in which the harms and benefits of any individual action must be weighed up such that a consideration of the benefits of lockdown orders is warranted, arguments often emerged to dismiss the lockdown as more harmful than the risk of spreading the virus – a point to which I will return below in the context of the perceived psychological harms of social isolation.

Additionally, a variant of the protest response involved the populism of the pre-existing 'sovereign citizen movement', which is a loose group of activists who tactically interpret common law and long-repealed statutes such as the English Magna Carta of 1215 to claim that they are not subject to laws they find unfavourable, including particularly criminal codes, taxation law, driver and vehicle registration requirements, sometimes using violence to assert their claims and other times frustrating the ordinary process of law and governance through belligerence (Matza 2020). Where the so-called 'Sov-Cits' refused to comply with restrictions on mobility and movement in North America, Europe, Australia and elsewhere, it was not the liberal-humanist perspective of a claim to the illegitimacy of the mandatory requirements themselves, but their perception of the illegitimacy of governments to make orders of any kind whatsoever. As the most sensationalist and most vocal part of the anti-lockdown protests in many jurisdictions, the Sov-Cit belligerence became the face of the disavowal of lockdown.

Other threads of protest discourse drew on conspiracy theories, such as the (absurd) idea that there was no virus, but that illness was a by-product of 5G mobile telephony towers or that false claims about a virus were being used by governments or a hidden 'deep state' to control citizens, including their movement (Cover, Haw and Thompson 2022: 81). Others, of course, were driven to protest due to seeing it as an opportunity to monetize dissent (Knaus 2022). Ironically, of course, public protests bring bodies together in an assembly of people-ness (Butler 2015) that, itself, is not only in defiance of the health measures but also produces the conditions for the further spread of the virus. While protests were covered regularly enough in news media around the world to cause alarm about the possibility of insurrection or the destabilization of governments, they of course did no such thing – protests have long been a built-in part of the expected response to unfavourable or unpopular legislation and executive orders, what Herbert Marcuse (1964: 25) described as the 'ceremonial part of practical behaviourism, its harmless negation … quickly digested by the status quo as part of its healthy diet'.

A third response framework was grounded in neither complete compliance nor dissent, but in the calculation of risk. In Chapter 1, I discussed some of the ways in which the public had been further exposed to a biopolitical discourse of population risk management during the pandemic (and I will return to the performativity of risk calculation when I discuss vaccines in Chapter 7). Some of the responses to lockdown, quarantine and isolation followed the same biopolitical frameworks in ways which disavow both the compliance and individualism frameworks outlined above, and instead were experienced through a plotting of one's behaviours in terms of biopolitics and risk. Rather than the norm/abnorm of discipline that early quarantine measures in European towns attempted to inculcate, biopolitics operates at an everyday level through normative distributional curves, whereby variance from a norm can be diverse – to a limit. As Foucault put it, certain distributions are considered to be 'more normal than the others, or at any rate more favorable than the others' (Foucault 2007: 63).

In this framework, we witnessed a risk assessment approach not related to decisions as to whether or not to *comply* with mandatory lockdowns, but in relation to the *extent* to which people tested its limits. Most people I know in Melbourne pushed the bounds of lockdown rules, either spending more than the one (or later two) hours allowed for outdoor exercise, visiting a friend during periods when home visits were banned or moving further than the distance limitation rules allowed. According to one report, 60 per cent of people in the UK knew at least one person who had broken the UK lockdown rules (Serco Institute 2022). Here it is not defiance of the rules, but a careful mapping of hazard (of infection), risk (of being caught), benefits (to mental well-being), advantages (to others, such as in delivering food to an elderly neighbour) and so on. By recognizing a counter-public discourse in which many admitted openly to 'bending rules', one plots out on a curve of normativity the extent to which one can be at variance with rules of immobility without necessarily defying them. In this context, a convergence of subjectivity, behaviour, space and the force of law form a complex matrix against which one maps the self as a 'good citizen'.

Mobility and identity

If the frameworks by which people managed the enforced immobility during lockdown periods ranged across compliance, disavowal and a more complex plotting of variance; and if the ethical and health benefits of lockdowns were broadly clear to the majority of people (Cadesky 2020), then in what ways can the restriction of mobility be understood to change or re-constitute practices of identity, subjectivity and selfhood? The starting point to making sense of how restricted movement impinges on everyday practices of identity is to apprehend *mobility itself* as an ordinary cultural practice of identity. Indeed mobility is the marker of the contemporaneity in contemporary society: ubiquitous, often desired, a structure of feeling that emerged in the last three decades of the twentieth century and from which there is no turning back (Urry 2007). This is the mobility of movement in cities in which we ourselves are part of the body-city assemblage (Grosz 1995); it is the mobility of travel for work and leisure; the movement of students to study at universities and colleges in locations remote from their homes; the ease of visitation among different households and across age-groups such as children regularly seeing grandparents in retirement homes and hospices; and of course the border crossings the norm of which is both ease for some populations, citizens and groups and restrictions for others such as the subject *sans papier* for whom neither mobility nor stillness is an option (Derrida 1999: 101).

Mobility is not, of course, *universal* – there are very substantial distinctions across, say, the figure of the middle-class *flâneur* moving about the city (Featherstone 2006: 594) or the travelling millennial influencer sharing images of a persistently liminal experience of space (Wyn and Woodman 2006: 496–7), the refugee in a camp or detention whereby their futural mobility is unknowable (Pugliese 2004: 299), the person with a physical disability living in an urban setting designed for walking up steps (Woodward 2002: 104) and those whose labour is marked by night-time mobility such as the drivers and cleaners who facilitate the free mobility of white-collar workers during the day (Sharma 2008: 462). Nevertheless, in each of these cases the performativity of a self-identity based on geographic location, pleasures, desires, consumption, labour, careers, minority communities and so on is marked and performed by varying degrees of mobility and movement.

If the performativity of identity is produced in the context of relational and social interdependency as an *a priori* fact of survival, as I have been arguing across previous chapters, then we need to acknowledge that one core element of interdependency is produced through mobility that enables access to the infrastructural supports that enable corporeal life – what Lauren Berlant (2016: 393) referred to as 'the living mediation of what organizes life: the lifeworld of structure'. In her assessment of interdependency, Butler hints at the ways in which mobility operationalizes access to the ecologies of infrastructure that support bodies to live:

> [T]he pavement is also an instrument for support, as are the traffic lights and the curb stops. It is not only those who are disabled who require support in order to move, to be fed, or indeed, to breathe. All of these basic human capacities are supported in one way or another. No one moves or breathes or finds food who is not supported by a world that provides an environment built for passage.
>
> (Butler 2020: 41)

In other words, movement through spaces via the conduits and technologies of mobility that society has constructed is at the core of our being. We perform our shared sense of humanity through movement, corporeal bodies shifting through space for survival, for comfort, for pleasure, for novelty. And even for those who cannot, we invest in the technologies to enable movement, whether wheelchairs or accessible pavements. And, finally, our performativity of selfhood is not divorced from our corporeality – it is 'acted out', as it were, through the movement of the body in space, in formations of proximity and distance from others, towards unknown spaces and back towards the familiarity of homes in ways which mark out our subjectivities as subjects who inhabit spaces and do so by the affective movement towards and back (Ahmed 1999: 341). None of this is to say that our experience of mobility and movement is equally enjoyed or even desired in the same way, but it is difficult to think about identity, sociality and belonging in contemporary culture without thinking about bodies coming and going through shared spaces.

Lockdown as disturbance of subjectivity

When mobility is the formation by which we are constituted as bodies – in space and in interdependency with other bodies – at both the ontological levels of corporeal survival and aesthetic, affective engagement with the familiar and the unfamiliar, to be restricted from mobility is to be ruptured as a subject. In other words, it is important not to fall into the epistemological trap of assuming that a restriction on mobility in the context of a pandemic lockdown is necessarily a constraint on some liberal concept of a 'natural' freedom of movement. Rather, the effect of the lockdown measures on a near-global scale foregrounds the ways in which, as subjects, we are constituted not merely in relationality with others on a planetary scale, but with the spaces we move through, desire to move through or are yet to move through as the mechanization of the performativity of interdependent relationality.

Important here is to recognize that, as subjects, we are constituted in our engagement with a spatial ecology that includes more than just the 'home' (for those who have it) and the 'familiar' (such as the streets of towns and cities in which we choose or are required to live, the places where one buys food). Rather, it includes the novel (the trip to somewhere new, the alternative route in a car home, a restaurant that one has never previously tried, a trip to a hospital for surgery for the first time). What does it mean, then, when the irreversible condition of being bodies cohabiting a spatial ecology in which movement is the customary and recurring practice of engagement with space is forcibly constrained such that 'at home' and 'the familiar', whether with family and housemates or physically alone, is the limitation of mobility? In what ways does this re-shape the ecology that constitutes us?

An ecology is usually defined as the mutual relations of organisms with their environment and with one another. We could take that a step further, as in anthropologist Margaret Mead's (1964) definition, an ecological setting includes the geographical, human and nonhuman groups that provide the conditions for sustainability and cultural evolution (148–9). If bodies are interdependent from the beginning – and they are – then that is an interdependency that is constituted within, through and emplaced by the geographical, conceptual and social ecologies that guarantee (for some) liveability. Within that practice of liveability, however, are two competing desires related to how we engage and are constituted by that ecology: the desire to be safe (from disease by restricting mobility) and the desire to be mobile (by performing selfhood in a wide array of spatial settings, including the novel). Arguably, we have here an incompatibility between those two practices that can be described as a 'chasm' at the very instance, in the context of the pandemic, we are asked to foreground making sense of it by conceptualizing what we cannot, be law, do. Here, the requirement to be safe (for ourselves, for humanity) by remaining relatively immobile, and the deep attachment to the cultural demand for social participation through mobility presents not a choice but an untranslatability that calls upon subjects to expend the anxious affective labour in negotiating. This is because the discourse by which safety through lockdown is framed as an ethical, biopolitical obligation is radically separate from the discourse by which performativity of the disciplined self is produced.

In normal circumstances, disciplinary and biopolitical power operate in compatibility, biopolitics emerged later than disciplinary frameworks, building upon it to extend its institutional practices of normalization and surveillance into the sphere of administration and governance (Foucault 2004a: 242). However, in the context of a *crisis* in which mobility itself becomes the object of power, discipline and biopolitics diverge: our disciplinary practices of mobility in order to conform to demands for social participation, labour and engagement and our biopolitical requirement to protect the population by remaining immobile present an incompatibility at the heart of the mutual operations of these power forms.

We can perceive, then, the pandemic-related operations of two separate discourses as being both framed by a monolingualism for which there is no assimilation or translation. Translation is, for Derrida (1978: 210), always impossible because it relies on an impossible fundamental capacity for signifiers to be substituted. Here, the ability to translate the two competing discourses around mobility establishes an abyss, whereby one discourse cannot be integrated into another without producing abjection and destabilization (Kristeva 1982: 14). Such an abyss is, for John Caputo (1993: 239), a destabilizing force:

> The abyss is just another name for what happens, for the happening of events, for the fact that events happen because they happen, cut off from the comforts of a deep and reassuring ground. The abyss is the decapitation of events, the loss of the Meta-event. But that can be disturbing.

In this respect, the competing desires or demands for mobility as fundamental to subjective being, on the one hand, and, on the other, the ethical demands of immobility for survival on the other present an aporia which calls upon the subject to find new constituting ground that can 'cope' with the abyss and incorporate it into subjectivity itself. Hope for a future of an end to lockdown was one particular re-constitutive force for many, marked by the celebrational cultural practice of 'freedom days' in many jurisdictions (Hui and Faulconbridge 2021) whereby the theatrics of an impending carnivalesque release puts the aporia on hold, making lockdown a liminality to be passed through.

Contra the psychological harms of lockdown

Regulated immobility was, during much of its time, discussed in terms of an imposition of *isolation*, which was to read isolation as being non-contact with the unfamiliar one encounters in ordinary mobility or with a wider group of people with whom one is not ordinarily 'at home'. I would like to consider here some of the ways in which a public sphere discourse framed mobility restriction health measures as an enforced isolation that, as was sometimes claimed, was harmful to the mental health of populations. This is an important consideration, because it is necessary to differentiate such claims from the framework of reconstitution I have presented above in which subject – on the whole – demonstrated a phenomenal capability of resilience in managing and navigating the competing needs of being a subject that is ordinarily and fundamentally constituted in mobility.

A number of political and protest arguments were put forward that claimed – often falsely – that the isolation of lockdowns was causing an unprecedentedly very high rate of suicides. In Australia, an open letter to the prime minister and premiers of Australian states from a group of 'concerned citizens' demanded an end to COVID-19 lockdowns on the basis of a range of harms, including 'rising suicide rates' (Joyce 2020). Several business leaders demanded an end to the Melbourne lockdown also on basis that it had increased suicides (Black 2020). Later that same year, Australian treasurer Josh Frydenberg used a speech in Parliament to criticize the lockdown measures in the state of Victoria, claiming a 'friend of a friend' had died by suicide 'due to lockdown' (Wren 2020). The actual suicide of a former Australian soap actor during a shorter lockdown in Sydney was widely used as a reason to criticize mobility restrictions (Piotrowki and Chain 2021). Finally, the Australian Christian Lobby called on the public to demand leaders 'fully restore freedoms' on the basis also of inaccurate claims about high suicide rates (ACL 2021). Similarly, in the United States, former president Donald Trump claimed from very early in the pandemic that any isolation restrictions that might impact the economy would lead to suicide numbers greater than the death toll from unfettered COVID-19 infections (Cathey 2020).

The reality was that the accusations that lockdowns were causing suicides were based on assumptions rather than genuine coronial data (which, rightly, lags behind events if deaths are to be properly investigated), but later proved to be completely incorrect (Pakman 2021). Indeed, the Coroner's office in the Australian state of Victoria, where one of the longest lockdowns was taking place, found no increase in the rate of completed suicides (The New Daily 2020) and, after a study of suicides that occurred during the period, found that while COVID-19 itself may have been an added stressor, the majority of suicides during the restriction periods were of subjects who had pre-existing mental health conditions (Tuohy 2021). In some Australian jurisdictions, suicide rates dropped during the mobility restriction era (Lifeline 2020; Clun 2021), although it is recognized that self-harming and non-suicidal mental health emergencies did increase substantially in some regions (Berger 2021).

Inaccurate suicide rate claims were thus used primarily as a political and protest tool to argue against regulatory immobility (Wren 2020). Nevertheless, almost a year after the final Melbourne lockdown, Stanford University epidemiologist Jay Bhattacharya – an avid opponent of lockdown measures and a co-author of the *Great Barrington* Declaration (2020) which raised public health concerns about COVID-19 policies – stated that he expected to see widespread 'psychological harms from lockdowns' in Melbourne (Le Grand 2022). Arguably, we may find that any evidence of psychological stresses result more from emerging from lockdowns into new forms of inequality than from the shared experience of lockdowns themselves.

Naturally, the myth of lockdown-caused suicidality shifted from arguments and assumptions into social media and circulated widely in the way that much disinformation ordinarily flows (Cover, Haw and Thompson 2022). Why, however, did the factually incorrect myth that mobility restrictions had caused high increases in suicide rates circulate so easily and believably among both those who were criticizing lockdowns and those who were reading these arguments in the press? The answer is that the believability in large numbers of suicides caused by mobility restrictions is grounded in a pre-existing 'suicide logic' (Kral 1994) that connects mobility restrictions with isolation, and isolation or loneliness with suicidality.

In the context of the first link, the conflation of mobility restrictions or stay-at-home orders with isolation or loneliness is highly problematic: while certain experiences of loneliness might indeed be understood in relation to certain ways of being that are perceived as unliveable, isolation was *not* the experience for many in lockdown. Rather, a substantial engagement with sociality was broadly at play at a range of levels. For example, in March 2020 when Italy was among the first countries to experience mobility restrictions, a great outpouring of communities singing together from balconies above deserted streets occurred in Naples and Rome (Horowitz 2020). Engagement with entertainment on streaming services increased dramatically such that ordinarily fragmented viewership merged into the older-style experience of the broadcast television era in which large segments of the population share the same entertainment (Maddox 2020). Group workshops, art classes and other activities were formed across Skype and Zoom online, engaging people who were otherwise more isolated before the pandemic (Topsfield 2020), while white-collar employees, business people and students following mandatory orders to remain at home engaged with each other on-screen to such an extent that 'zoom fatigue' from extensive meetings and online social engagement became a new issue for many (Chrisoulakis 2021).

Finally, rather than isolation and social fragmentation, we might also say that the experience of widespread lockdowns – on both city and global scales – was one of very substantial *shared experience*: the knowledge that we are not experiencing a phenomenon alone but that our immobility is shared to the point that reporting significant breaches became a cultural practice (Koob and Butt 2020) not because it was a breach of rules but a breach of the shared sociality of immobility. It is, of course, inaccurate to state that no one was isolated or lonely, or that there was no stress and anxiety for those living in crammed conditions, in poorly ventilated or poorly heated homes, in persistently noisy conditions, or in stressful family situations, or living alone without the prospect of physical touch and proximity to other subjects, or being among the front-line health workers who were required to face daily risks when immobility might be preferable. However, the common parlance of the health restrictions as 'isolation' not only demonstrates the core mobility at the heart of interdependent sociality, but also presents a narrow view of how social engagement is performed today in ways which do not necessarily always demand movement and mobility.

The second link – isolation and suicide – likewise relies on a pre-existing cultural logic. Isolation in the form of *social disconnection* has long been recognized as a causal factor in suicidality, although as I am arguing here, mobility restrictions are not completely assimilable to social disconnection, broadly speaking. Emile Durkheim's (1952) studies of suicide in the late nineteenth century present a number of ways in which suicide can be thought differently from the prevailing suicidology frameworks of individualized mental health and depression and the pathologization of suicidal subject (White et al. 2016). Durkheim identified several approaches to making sense of suicides in terms of structures of communities in an attempt to explain why suicides were statistically fewer among members of highly cohesive religious societies (123–4). He developed a concept of 'egoistic suicide' which found suicidality was more likely to occur when individuals perceived themselves as individualized and isolated from a strong, well-integrated social community. He argued that the less *integrated* the society the more likely the suicide – social integration thereby operated as a preventative measure against suicidality (124–5). Here, 'excessive individuation' (167–9) and a detachment from society is a detachment from life itself since, in his formulation, a good life is a life directed *towards* society as both life's source and life's aim (170). The distress caused by a self-perception of non-integration or the lack of a cohesive social collectivity produces a disposition of unliveability through a melancholy that results from this 'same exaggerated individualism' (Durkheim 1952, 172–3). While Durkheim's suicide theories are no longer considered necessarily relevant to the twenty-first century, they carried such mythic weight during much of the twentieth century that a misperception of isolation as individuation was seen as a likely cause of suicides (Cover 2020c). Other authors working on the fringes of suicidology have, more recently, reiterated the isolation-suicide link. Thomas Joiner (2005), for example, articulated the notion of 'thwarted belonging' as one causality of suicide. For Joiner (2005: 117), isolation is experienced by the person who remains 'absolutely unnoticed' by fellow members of society, what we might re-frame as a sensibility of non-belonging in which a subject feels one is not 'listened to' (Dreher 2009) and thereby not recognized as a subject in the sense of belonging *to* sociality (Butler 2004: 44). Both Durkheim and Joiner's accounts of isolation have value in the sense of pointing to social disconnection as a framework of causality that can produce the kinds of identity breakdown in which suicide becomes the logical option to escape the intolerable emotional pain of social disconnectivity (Shneidman 1985: 36). However, when social disconnection and isolation due to immobility are not the same thing, it is necessary not to fall into the trap of assuming that physical isolation or restricted mobility is, in itself, a social disconnection – and instead necessary to see how the shared experience may well be a liveable one.

Indeed, not only is physical isolation and stillness considered a factor in the resilience and well-being of subjects (Cover 2020c), but we may consider how that social sharing of lockdown and the shared experience of the difficult labour of navigating re-constituted subjectivity and identity may be a protective factor against suicide and an explanation for why suicide rates not only did not rise but fell in some jurisdictions. One model of suicide causality derived from statistical findings and sociological research may well provide a useful way in which to understand how the shared experience of lockdown and immobility protects against suicide. James Barber (2001) criticized researchers and public commentators who discuss suicide in terms of *whole populations* in crisis. He referred to this depiction as the Absolute Misery Hypothesis, the 'intuitively straightforward notion that the suicide rate of a generation is a surrogate measure of that generation's happiness. The more suicides, the greater the level of unhappiness' (Barber 2001: 49). That is, economic disadvantage or discrimination against an *entire* community or society is erroneously assumed to result in a greater number of suicides, whereas cross-national analysis indicates that this has not always been the case – indeed, higher rates of suicide have been associated with higher levels of psychological adjustment, happiness and affluence among groups or whole populations (Smalley, Scourfield and Greenland 2005: 138). Barber countered the Absolute Misery Hypothesis with a proposal he termed the Relative Misery Hypothesis:

> According to the 'relative misery hypothesis', young men's predisposition to suicide is influenced by their social comparisons. When those around them are perceived to be better off than they are, the distress of vulnerable youth is magnified and their susceptibility to suicidality increased. The relative misery hypothesis would therefore predict a rise in suicide rates whenever there is a rise in the overall mood or happiness of a population, whether that rise is due to the end of war or any other event of general and positive social significance. At such times, the misery of the community's unhappiest young men will be compounded by the isolation they experience at witnessing the happiness of those around them.
>
> (Barber 2001: 53)

What Barber's framework points to is that the 'absolute misery' of a population – its shared experience of crisis, catastrophe, war, deprivation or, in this case, immobility and restrictions on some pleasurable forms of sociality, is not in itself indicative of higher suicide rates, but serves as a protective factor because it is broadly a shared experience. It is in emerging from the shared experience of immobility that relativity comes back into play: those who came out without employment, or lost homes, or suffered relationship breakdowns, or suffered psychological harms or other disadvantages relative to their peers who thrived. Restricted mobility here is not only something we cannot necessarily call isolation, but the sense of isolated and social disconnectedness emerges after the shared experience is over when some emerge with a sense of stability and others do not. The extent, then, to which our access to the infrastructural supports of the ecologies in which we survive and perform sociality through mobility is equitable is a key issue in how we might better perceive the good or the harms of health restrictions based on mobility restrictions.

Conclusion

What the experience of corporeal life during the unfinished pandemic years has highlighted is our attachment to mobility as a foundational kernel of subjectivity wrought in interdependency not only with others but with the supportive and infrastructural ecology that is accessed in terms of space and the social and physical technologies that enable us to traverse it. Our radical, deep dependency on infrastructures that enable the movement of food, the provision of electricity, the requirement of shelter and the necessity of medical care, science and digital networks for communication has thereby drawn out and made apparent our corporeal interdependency without which survival is not an option. Once we think about subjectivity, mobility and the spatiality of infrastructural ecologies together, we can recognize that our performativity through movement in space and both into and away from contact with one another is tenuous, precarious formation by which we simultaneously encounter pleasure (one another), survival (access to the corporeal supports of life), as well as risk (of disease and harm).

This fact, thereby, opens up onto the field of violence and ethics – an important consideration given the failure to comply with mobility restrictions during a pandemic is an act of violence to those we may never meet but whose life may be lost should we unwittingly spread the virus to them. Violence never exhausts itself in the perpetration of an act or injury, but always exceeds its instrumentalism and intent (Butler 2020: 19–20). At the same time, then, adopting a counter-discourse that perceives immobility as a harm or restraint, rather than as a re-positioning of subjectivity, is foreclosed on the possibility of considering our relationship with each other and the spatial, infrastructural ecology in ways which may lead towards a more ethical way of doing mobility in the future.

5

Disrupted exposure: Ethics and the face of the other in the time of masks

Introduction

During much of the long 2021 lockdowns experienced in Melbourne, my partner and I were fortunate to spend much of it at our house in country Victoria. We had long planned to split our time between the city and country, an ideal escape from urban noise, a place to write in solitude and a setting for respite from the routine of work without the carbon footprint of air travel that had marked so much of our lives until 2020. When an earlier lockdown ended so that we could finally collect the keys to a place we had bought but not seen for several months, we had never envisaged that this house on the outskirts of a small country town would become a long-term refuge after being banned from crossing back into the city for several months. However, rural area restrictions were far lighter than those of the city (perhaps a little unfairly) and this meant some greater freedoms to enjoy movement and fresh air, albeit within a fairly tight radius from home.

While walking back one afternoon from the town's green-grocer, we were confronted by an elderly woman – not a local, as we later discovered – who screamed at us for wearing our N95 (also known as P2) masks: 'take them off! take them off! COVID's all a hoax!' and tried to pull the mask from my face. Shocked, we walked away hurriedly saying nothing, but were followed as the woman tried repeatedly to remove our masks. In the following months we occasionally heard similar stories, although almost all others occurred in the context of a confrontation between COVID-denying protesters and bystanders who engaged them. The incident, however, was eye-opening: a practice of mask-wearing that had become *normative to us* was not viewed in the same way by others who found masks on other people's faces to be, itself, threatening and confronting. For us, of course, this was also an assault: an attempt to forcibly remove an item of clothing would be considered not merely a breach of etiquette but, in many jurisdictions, a likely crime. It was a moment of realization at how much the mask had become an intimate part of clothing in everyday public life – the attempt to rip it off being about as violating as an attempt to forcibly remove another person's clothing. Finally, of course, it was an instance of being made to feel vulnerable – as the mask pulled away from my mouth, the realization that the perpetrator's breath and fingers were uncomfortably close to my nose and mouth (although of course not much closer than we might have experienced on a crowded train without concern only a couple of years earlier). Again, an instance of awareness at the extent to which the mask had become not only a piece of essential safety equipment, but also an object of controversy and sometimes aggression.

Masks were already a matter of heated debate, of course, once it became clear that SARS-CoV-2 was transmitted in aerosolized droplets from breath. Donald Trump denounced face coverings as a form of protection on many occasions and even when pushed to encourage its use gave mixed messages about their utility (Victor, Serviss and Paybarah 2020). Masks became a symbol of the pandemic, an object of both dependency and derision among people with polarized attitudes, and in an everyday sense a material artefact that, in Western countries unused to masking during periods of illness, became suddenly a cultural form and practice, an item of identity disruption as well as an item of identity performativity. The figure of the face mask since it was introduced as a pandemic health measure sits then at the intersection of competing attitudes, ethics, formations of subjectivity and politics.

In this chapter, I would like to address three ways in which the mask – as a form of communication in itself – intersects with our cultural practices of identity. Following a brief summary of the introduction of the mask into everyday life in parts of the world where its use has been rare, I discuss how the obscuring of people's faces can be understood in terms of ethics, drawing on and re-thinking Emmanuel Levinas' ethics of non-violent responsibility based on the exposure to the face of others. I will then work through some of the ways in which the mask has been reacted to differentially, particularly in terms of its perception as an object of vulnerability and/or weakness before discussing some of the problematic practices in which anti-maskers have been shamed and how that act of shaming has operated as a problematic performance of identity. I will conclude with some remarks on how the corporeal normativization of the mask for the wider majority who adopted it can be apprehended as a disruptive-adjustment of identity performativity itself.

The emergence of the mask and polarized debates

Deborah Lupton and colleagues (2021) have provided an excellent analysis of the mask in the COVID years, addressing its role not merely as a health measure utilized in reducing transmission but as a socio-material object that has become not only part of everyday sociality, but also a key symbol of the pandemic given its use in regular news and entertainment images all over the world. They also point out the ways in which the mask has come to stand in for all sorts of contentions, as a visual symbol of the pandemic itself, and as an object that framed our experiences of engaging with others during a substantial period of time in the COVID years. I do not wish to repeat their powerful, systemic analysis, but to consider some of the ways in which mask-wearing emerged as a cultural controversy.

Face masks were an atypical health protection for most people living in Western countries, where masks are mostly associated with serious hospitalization, sometimes worn by hospital visitors during outbreaks of communicable illnesses such as staph infections, and occasionally associated with radical, paranoid 'survivalist' and 'prepper' behaviours (Poynting et al. 2004: 212). In a more aesthetic sense, the idea of masks more broadly has been associated in the West with 'play' including in the contexts of dressing up, parties, theatre and festivals in which we are separated from the everydayness of the exposed face (Huizinga 1949: 13). In this sense, the donning of masks as a health protection device has a slightly surreal sense to it – one of the most serious and necessary health measures during the pandemic and yet an act most of us had only ever associated with the fun of dressing up or disguise. And, of course, at a more philosophic level, the concept of the mask is strongly associated with suspicion, whether that is the masked criminal as the cliché bank robber, or the use of the metaphor of the mask as disguising hegemony, falsity, surreptitious values or inequalities as everyday concepts such as liberty, good governance or care (McCoy 1993: 147).

For those in East Asia and other parts of the world, the use of face masks was more common, recognizable and normative during regular seasons of illness – either to prevent contraction of an illness among the sensibly cautious or as a medical requirement to prevent spreading a virus while still infectious (Ma and Zhan 2022). They were also regularly used to avoid breathing pollutants, particularly in the streets during periods of smog or haze caused by fires in nearby countries. Indeed, for the past two decades, it has never been 'strange' to me to see people wearing masks on public transport in East Asian cities, but a rare event to see a face mask worn by anyone in London, New York, Sydney or most of continental Europe. The discrepancy in regional experience here is important, as from the very beginning of conceptualizing the use of face masks as a health measure, there is already an identity component to their use and the preparedness to adopt during the COVID years.

Finally, it should be noted that the discrepancy over practices of covering parts of the face is made more fraught by cultural differences that have been the subject of controversy, attempted regulation and violence, including particularly the wearing of the burqa, hijab or other forms of Islamic head-covering by migrants in some Western countries since the 11 September 2001 World Trade Center terrorist attack, and the years of war in Iraq and Afghanistan. This includes particularly France, where headscarves and other garments covering the face that are related to religious practice were banned in 2004 (Abdelgadir and Fouka 2020), and in Australia where debates over the wearing of a burqa into government buildings was a focus of far-right political parties for many years (9News 2017).

Although there had been a longer history of mask-wearing during the outbreak of infectious diseases, including in China since the early 1900s (Lynteris 2018), they were not initially recommended by the World Health Organization or most governments for use by healthy, non-infected people. Indeed, in late March, the World Health Organization recommended their use only by those in close contact with someone infected, and the same month the US surgeon general asked people not to buy masks. At the time the Czech Republic and some other countries had begun mandating masks early in the pandemic, the WHO perspective was grounded in a concern that masks would offer a false sense of security, would be worn incorrectly and that widespread purchase would take supply away from medical staff and those who need them for close contact with the infected (Lacina 2020). However, by the third quarter of 2020, more than one hundred jurisdictions had required their populations to use masks in public settings, and in those which did not make masks mandatory, many businesses were requiring customers and visitors to wear masks if they enter the indoor premises. Full mandates became more widespread by October 2020 when it was better recognized that SARS-CoV-2 was carried in aerosolized particles that could travel more widely than most social distancing limitations, rather than larger droplets that have a limited range (Lupton et al. 2021: 35, 47–8). At this point, the mask became a key preventative mechanism to reduce infection.

The introduction of the mask was, of course, problematic not in terms of the reaction from the public but of what amounted to a reversal of policy. While the concept of a mask in Western countries had moved by then from being seen as an ordinary object of play, of professional medical settings or of suspicion, the reversal on policy at both the World Health Organization and across many governments that followed WHO recommendations was seen as problematic. In a media sphere in which governments are regularly held to account for policy flip-flops, changes in approach or reversals of strategy, the mandating of masks was apprehended as suspicious, then, for a new reason: the routine alignment of 'integrity', 'honesty' and 'authenticity' with temporal consistency meant that those governments, authorities, businesses and health communicators who reversed position on masks were misrecognized as inauthentic. While obviously the majority of people in jurisdictions mandating the wearing of masks complied and understood the reasoning behind the change in policy, the spectre of inconsistency fuelled some of the refusal, protest and outrage among anti-maskers, leaving the relationship between mask-wearing and normative identity less stable than might otherwise have been desired.

Masks and the ethics of the face

If we are to consider from a cultural and philosophic standpoint what masks do for identity in the COVID years, we need to recognize the disruption to certain dominant Western practices and expectations of the exposure of the face as a normative part of identity performance and inter-relational belonging. Indeed, having the full face on display is not merely a matter of identification, such as making it difficult for a person who needs to identify us visually for a transaction to ensure we are the same person shown on our photographic ID cards. Rather, the questions around the visibility of the face operate at the intersection of cultural norms, performativity through facial visibility and expression, and the ethics of belonging in a society in which facial recognition forms part of social participation and engagement.

A common response around much of the world in the first few weeks of mandated mask-wearing was about personal discomfort, particularly involving tips and tricks to prevent glasses fogging up, to wear masks without gaps, to manage skincare and make-up, to enliven our look with distinctive patterns, and so on (Lupton et al. 2021). Another strand of discourse, however, was about the obscured face, with remarks such as that the layers of fabric between two people were giving some a feeling of being detached and not seeing the full face of the person they were speaking resulting in 'a loss of personal connection' (Tuohy 2020). Of course, many soon found that concerns about not being able to see a smile were unfounded as an adjustment took place that involved realizing a mask did less to obscure the display of emotion on a face than imagined (Aubrey 2020). Nevertheless, unease over the partial obscuring of the face has remained a key issue in public discourse since the introduction of mandatory mask-wearing.

Aspects of this complaint about masks related to the fact that obscuring the face disrupted a basic framework of everyday identity – whether that is the act of proving identity through documents containing a photo, a machine using facial-recognition software or the act of communicating with others with an open face. In many respects, the argument was often given on the basis that while mask-wearing became an essential health measure to reduce transmission of the virus, it was to be seen as an unfortunate disruption to the practice of identity because it obscured that most essential feature of the performance of selfhood: the face. There is, however, a somewhat more complex way in which to understand the centrality of the face in the visual performances of interdependent social belonging, and for that we can turn to philosopher Emmanuel Levinas.

For Levinas (1969), the encounter with the face of another is the site of an ethical relation in which subjects are called upon to respond, recognize and offer an obligation to the other. In Levinasian ethics, this recognizes the fact that we are from the beginning of life part of human sociality and this presents a primary responsibility towards the other whom we encounter face-to-face (Secomb 2007: 59). In this respect, the needs of the other are figured as taking priority over our own needs – one is obliged by virtue of being a subject 'to apprehend the Other's material needs and put those needs first' (Butler 2006: 127). The subject is summoned by the other to assume responsibility for the other's welfare without recompense or reciprocity precisely because this ethical demand precedes our formation as subjects in face-to-face encounters. In Levinas' approach to ethics, however, that face-to-face encounter is more than merely a metaphor for the ethical obligation to others, place, ecologies or the world. Levinas differentiated between the parties face-to-face and the 'third', being the faceless others with whom we are in a political relation and with whom we do not have that same ethical relationship – a point of criticism raised by later philosophers concerned that the face-to-face encounter is reified over obligations to others unknown and unseen (e.g. Butler 2012).

In a purely Levinasian perspective, then, obscuring the face can be understood as obscuring the foundation of the ethical relation on which our very identities are built. What we owe to the other in their otherness is disrupted because we cannot see the face fully, and this implies at a philosophic level the potential breakdown of the ethical relation which can, although different from the political and social relations through which we perform our subjectivity, imply the breakdown of the ethical conduct in sociality and politics (Raffoul 1998). In other words, this implies an interruption to how we perform our identities because we are not obliged (ethically) or normativized (politically and socially) to enact care to the other that overrides our own care. More recent revisions of Levinasian ethics take the encounter with the face as a metaphor for the primordial vulnerability of the other – the uncovered, most naked part of the body (Plant 2011: 57) which stands in for the vulnerability of others as embodied, corporeal subjects with whom we must engage in an ethics of non-violence (Butler 2012: 56). Nevertheless, the spectre of the face as pivotal in the primary instance of an ethical relation has lingered, and points to the everydayness with which we expect an ethical relationship to be one which begins with an open face seen and displayed. Naturally, such revisions that read Levinas' use of the face as problematic recognize that the corporeal vulnerability we share as embodied subjects exceeds the face, which can be non-visible to us or non-proximate without disrupting the obligation of ethics grounded in hospitality, care and non-violence (Butler 2012). That is, a mask may disrupt the view of faces in an adjustment of sociality and identity, but not necessarily producing a change in the ethical obligations to others.

Indeed, from such a perspective, it is worth remarking how the obligation to the other can be seen to play out in regard to our obligations to the person not wearing a mask. Although there has been substantial anger towards those who refuse masks and a practice of shaming those either for refusing or for failing to wear the mask correctly (a point I discuss in more detail below), such anger and shaming may in itself be unethical in the perspective on ethics described above. This is not because our faces may be obscured while theirs are open and apparent in an encounter with a non-masked subject. Rather, such an ethics acknowledges that the other is always produced in radical alterity or difference from ourselves. This involves understanding that the difference of the other cannot be subsumed by our own experiences, understandings, practices or preferences (Secomb 2007: 61). In this respect, while social normativization of mask-wearing during periods in which transmission of the virus may be fatal to others presents an obligation to ourselves to wear a mask so as not to harm the other (including the other whose face we have never seen and will never know), we cannot as individual subjects place the demand on the other to wear a mask, even if it places us at risk. We are bound to that other, no matter how dangerous their unmasked face might be to us, and while we may choose not to be around them, and while we may belong to a polity that demands they wear a mask, the obligation is not upon us to shame them or harm them for failing to wear a mask or to wear one correctly. This is not to suggest that a care rooted in a pedagogical relation with the other is wrong, or that advising with care is unethical, only that to make the demand or to use the violence of language, categorization, marginalization and othering of those who refuse the mask is unethical. Ethics is always a quandary and not a rule, and it is an opening for a way of performing a relationship with the other that starts with non-violence. Their exposed face may, in this sense, be unethical, but it is equally unethical to attempt to represent the polity or sociality by demanding the mask of them.

Identity and the corporeal normativization of the mask

Even if the diversity in mask-wearing practices to which we are obliged ethically sits uneasily against the desire for a normative adoption of masks during periods of high-risk social transmission of the virus, the debates in popular communication and everyday discourse about masks shift in the practice of identity. As Lupton and colleagues (2021: 49) neatly put it: 'Placing a mask on our face is deeply corporeal, sensory, and affective. It disrupts our usual ways of being in the world and reconfigures our relations with others'. This is an important consideration, and certainly one which shows the significance of temporality and stabilization to our practices of identity as many of us became 'used to' wearing a mask. Indeed, there is enough anecdotal evidence to suggest many people felt 'naked' once the mask was no longer needed or mandated in public. Why? Not only because the mask became normativized and an adjustment and incorporation occurred, but because it became very much a part of identity performativity in the context of the pandemic.

The mask is not simply something that overlays upon or obscures our identity; an inconvenience or a tool that we willingly embrace. Rather, masks intersect with the performance of identity in multiple ways, including ways which perform and identify ourselves as conforming to a group norm. As a marker of identification, the mask plays a key role by indicating in our performance of wearing it a range of attitudes and beliefs to others. This is not to suggest that identifying with a normative practice is fully aligned with all beliefs and attitudes – rather multiple identifications are always possible, such as identifying with and practising the norm of wearing a mask while questioning their utility as a protection against COVID, feeling that mandatory requirements to wear masks are wrong, or indeed having multiple opinions. As Diana Fuss (1995: 49) notes, identity always involves negotiating with multiple and competing identifications that produce 'conflicts to be managed'. The management of those conflicting identifications is likely to have been a far more common – and often exhausting – experience among the vast majority who wore masks. In other words, adopting mask-wearing was not simply a matter of obedience or willing and enthusiastic adoption of a shift in identity practices, but a *negotiation* that demanded the labour of incorporating, adjusting and stabilizing.

At the same time, wearing a mask or not wearing a mask serves as an identifier of affiliation. We are, as biopolitical subjects, called upon to position ourselves on a distributional curve of normativities in ways which are proximate with the norm – the extent to which we wear a mask, wear it well, keep it on, take breaks in settings in which we should not, and so on is about that negotiated positioning, and in many ways this is non-voluntarist and often without conscious agency. Those who refuse the mask outright and disobey the mandates too are performing in a particular way involving affiliation and identification, particularly in the context of media representations of polarized views on mask-wearing that often excluded the reality of a normative curve and diverse engagement with the practice. This, of course, does not exclude mis-identification and mis-recognition of identities in relation to the wearing of masks, as well as the perception that one might be misrecognized: for example, in having forgotten to wear a mask (as many of us did in unfortunate slippages) and be accidentally identified as anti-maskers.

Again, without wanting to eschew the significance of a profound diversity of experiences, at a philosophic level it is possible to remark that the face mask is incorporated as an aspect of the performativity of identity. As Butler (1991) has noted, the repetition of a particular way of performing the self stabilizes and reconstitutes the self over time. That is not to suggest that in the very act of repetition the inherent instability of subjectivity is always at play, but to say that in the context of change and disruption, we smooth over those identity instabilities by performing *as if* always stable and linear. Where obscuring the face with a mask was, for many, a new and unusual and unsettling experience, and for some an act that could never be incorporated into their everyday lives, for many others it was a practice that was not only normativized but became actively incorporated in a corporeal way into a stable identity to 'feel natural'. Just as for many people (not all), our genders, our racial identities or ethnicities and other facets of identity come to seem 'natural' over time – even if such natural feeling is always from the beginning an illusion – so too did the act of wearing a mask, of being identified as a 'mask wearer' and of performing those identities under the surveillance of others.

Masks and vulnerability

If our identity is constituted in a primary vulnerability, since as corporeal subjects we are always vulnerable and share that vulnerability, then it is useful to consider how the different registers of vulnerability through which masks have been discussed has played out. Indeed, the very idea of the mask is entwined with concepts of vulnerability, whether worn or not. Vulnerability is, as we know from Butler's (2004) extensive work on the topic, a primary aspect of corporeal life that is closely entwined with how our subjectivity is formed from the very beginning in interdependency with others. In one very key respect, our very survival as individualized subjects depends to some extent on others recognizing our mutual vulnerability to the virus, and on their wearing masks as we wear masks, doubly protecting from potential transmission. And certainly the site of masks on large numbers of people operated as a reminder of our own vulnerability to disease and the vulnerability of others (Lupton et al. 2021: xiii), particularly given the greater visual presence of masks in both the streets and on screens in the latter parts of the pandemic while mortality and hospitalization rates were presented not in visuals but in the more clinical form of statistics and graphs.

However, mask-wearing has been associated with other registers of vulnerability that are not so much part of that primary vulnerability we all share as corporeal subjects. Rather, these are registers that are wholly separate from that primary vulnerability whereby vulnerability is conceived as differential and as experienced unevenly and undemocratically distributed depending on a host of identity-based criteria, from age to socio-economic status to racial background (and especially in many parts of the world, to Indigeneity). In this respect, the significance of wearing a mask not only is about normativity, conformity or stabilized as part of embodied identity as a norm, but also involves differential *tactics* that enable survival, and are among the many tactics that the oppressed and marginalized must adopt on a day-to-day basis (Bhabha 1994). In some ways, those tactics can include the need to make a choice not to wear a mask in order to enable other forms of support and belonging, thereby positioning certain subjects to *calculate* and *weigh up* competing vulnerabilities in ways which are disregarded by the universal media messaging around mandatory and recommended mask-wearing.

A second register of the vulnerability of mask-wearing is more cynical – the act of associating masks with 'weakness'. This has been widely recognized as a mark of President Trump's response to masks, his ridiculing of his political opponents for wearing masks and the framing of masks as non-vigorous and effeminate (Lupton et al. 2021: 38, 74). In this context, wearing a mask is seen not as a recognition of corporeal vulnerability to disease, but as marking a distinction between vigour and bravado on the one hand and care, weakness and fear on the other. It is, of course, no accident that simplistic approaches such as this have a tendency to frame a complex issue through dichotomies that align with masculine/feminine gender binaries. Such approaches to gender and their deployment as frameworks to understand complex social issues draw on older, outdated notions of masculinity that align it with strength, national interest and risk (Connell 1995, Wheaton 2000) pitted against an 'other' which, in this case, is perceived as fear and self-inflicted or unnecessary vulnerabilization – thereby missing the point that such dichotomies have always been overly simplistic (Beasley 2008). Here, a particular approach to mask-wearing aligns identity, gender and the performance of wearing a mask as an identity grounded in shame in ways which are the converse from the earlier shaming of anti-maskers described above. This is not to suggest that this is polarized, but to point out that part of the reaction to mask debates has required people to navigate more than just protection from disease but also the multiple registers through which vulnerability is perceived, together creating new cultural formations of identity performance and belonging.

There is also an interesting twist on vulnerability in which those who know better and have worn masks have also ceased wearing them and made themselves vulnerable to infection. In my own city, we witnessed this in November 2020 after a protracted period of diligent compliance with mandatory mask-wearing while attempting to pursue a zero-infection policy. On a public holiday, social isolation regulations were breached when thousands of residents spent the day at St Kilda beach, most not wearing masks – substantial footage was shown across the country of unusually festive behaviour, including defying long-standing bans on drinking alcohol, while public dance parties started up in nearby parks (Dexter and Pearson 2020). Naturally, the administrative response was that this behaviour put at risk the work towards keeping infections low in the pre-vaccination era.

Foucault (2004b: 47) identified a literary trend that described a practice during plague periods in the sixteenth and seventeenth centuries in which members of a population abandoned fear and a sense of vulnerability to throw off their metaphorical 'identity' masks in mass behaviours of debauchery, lawlessness and collective risk. Here, a re-framing of identity through abandonment of protective measures is celebrated as a political act that topples regulatory measures in favour of abandonment. While the conditions that encourage people to embrace the vulnerabilization of the self by dropping all protective behaviours and taking on the risk of transmission differ substantially between the seventeenth and twenty-first centuries, the parallel is indicative of the way in which the collective refusal operates within a disjuncture in ordinary identity practices that incorporate the management of risk. Here, we see the practice of identity in singularity subsumed by a collective subjectivity of the kind seen in other festive and carnival temporalities (Cover 2013b). In this context, the mask represents neither protection nor vulnerability, but the singularity of identity – despite the practice of wearing it being itself part of the performance of identity through the frame of belonging, compliance and normativization. Such a reversal in behaviour is not *about* the mask (or the other protective measures such as social distancing), but about the carnivalesque abandonment of subjectivity that establishes the norms by performing the abandonment of the norm.

Conclusion

Face masks, then, can be understood as being part of a complex assemblage of new cultural practices, calling upon subjects not only to manage the adaptation to and incorporation of masks into everyday corporeal subjectivity, as well as the irritation, unfamiliarity and change. Rather, the demand has been to negotiate and manage the ethical implications (how to respond to the other if the face is no longer fully visible), the identity implications (how to incorporate and manage self-identity when the practice of doing so is disrupted by a new necessity) and the cultural implications (the different registers by which masks are framed as markers of vulnerability). The serious implications that emerge when the refusal to wear a mask puts others – perhaps ourselves – at risk while an ethical perspective demands that we not shame or disavow the anti-masker adds to that complexification.

If, as I argue across this book, the key 'learning' that must be made from the experience of COVID-19 is that we are subjects of diverse interdependency and must disavow individualist thinking to survive a dangerous virus, then part of that practice of interdependency is recognizing the sheer complexity required to be ethical. Drawing from the Levinasian perspective described above, we must offer hospitality and non-violence to those others with whom we are interdependent, which means wearing masks to protect from the transmission of the virus through our breath that is shared by virtue of being interdependent in proximity, but at the same time not inflicting the violence of shaming on those who do not. Learning to navigate the array of conflicting demands produced by mask-wearing as a health protection is an important, necessary step to getting something out of the inconvenience of masking up.

6

Disrupted touch: Hands, bodies and social distancing

Introduction

When the COVID-19 pandemic first began to have an impact in the United States, a number of early measures were taken to reduce the spread of the virus by encouraging social distancing. The intervention taken in the state of Florida was an order by Governor Ron DeSantis to shut down bars and nightclubs for thirty days, directions to require beach gatherings of no more than ten people with a minimum of six feet distance between groups and a reduction in the patronage of restaurants to fifty per cent capacity (State of Florida 2020). The measures drew on Centers for Disease Control and Prevention (CDC) guidelines early in the pandemic to limit contact and touch between human beings in order to prevent spread. This was considered to be a particularly significant practice at the time, as, although it was suspected in the first half of 2020 that SARS-CoV-2 was transmitted through airborne, aerosolized particles, this was not formally recognized by the World Health Organization until October 2020 (Lewis 2022a). This meant that keeping bodies from touching each other, or touching surfaces in the environment where the virus may have been shed, was understood as the best mechanism to prevent transmission (World Health Organization 2022). Reducing crowds and keeping bodies apart, in other words, was the principal weapon in preventing the spread of COVID-19 in the early months.

The governor's executive order coincided with the start of the March–April Spring Break period, when very large crowds of students holiday at Miami beaches, attending massive parties and festivals, particularly in Florida settings such as Panama City Beach, Fort Lauderdale and Miami Beach. News coverage of those settings broadcast interviews with many young people disappointed to have their festivities spoiled and objecting to the closure of bars and clubs. Others, however, spoke in defiance of the social distancing orders, unwilling to suspend their partying to avoid the risk of transmission. One young man became globally known for his statement of defiance when his brief sound-byte circulated the globe through news and social media: 'If I get corona, I get corona. At the end of the day, I'm not going to let it stop me from partying' (Bella 2020).

There were, of course, a number of factors as to why young party-goers were not taking it seriously, including then President Trump's playing down of the significance of the pandemic and the perception that young people were at much less risk of becoming severely unwell. Although the young man was widely mocked, and later apologized publicly for his arrogance and assumptions of his invincibility (Ortiz 2020), this particular instance provided an important impetus for public debate on the ethics of touch and prompted a deeper public introspection into the ways in which touch, bodies-in-proximity and contact among crowds provide the framework of interdependency through which viral transmission is likely. That is, what the young man later recognized in apologizing particularly to elderly people is that the touch, proximity and contact among a group of young people partying have a direct relationship with other forms of touch, including hugging a grandparent who may be at risk of death as a result of the physical contact he might make at a Spring Break festival.

This chapter addresses some of the issues related to touch and proximity of bodies that emerged across the pandemic, with a view to understanding how transmission sheds a light on the practices and norms of touch. Whether in the context of lockdowns and restricted mobility, or during periods of movement and gathering, many jurisdictions around the world encouraged, advised or enforced practices of social distancing which in one respect was recognized through regulation of immobilities as I discussed in Chapter 4. In another respect, this was a practice of intervention in the complex area of proximities of bodies (nearly touching; actually touching) which produced certain shifts in how we utilize touch, closeness and proximity as forms of community and as shared cultural practices of identity, subjectivity and belonging. Questions of touch also open the possibility to critique concepts of 'staying in touch' that do not involve physical proximity, and what it means to belong to communities and societies when visual practices of communication replace those of physical proximity and closeness.

I would therefore like to begin by discussing some of the practices of touch that signify greeting, acceptance, agreement and belonging in sociality, and how they changed in the context of social distancing regulations and recommendations. I will then turn to how touch and proximity operate in forms of identity performance, oscillating across communication and vulnerability. This is followed by a discussion of 'staying in touch' and how some of the ways in which this was visually experienced speak not merely to what was 'lost' but the fact that practices of affection, agreement and social bond are more diverse than the cultural norms or customs of touch represent. I would like to end with a brief discussion of proximity in the context of crowded spaces, which has a separate, long history of critique that, itself, urgently shifted in the context of the pandemic.

Namaste

For many of us around the world, social distancing practices remained a key component in the array of measures deployed to prevent the spread of the disease, from reduced numbers in theatres and limitations on the number of people permitted simultaneously in shops; from queue-markers outside bakeries requiring people to stand more than a metre apart, to less-conscious practices of keeping a distance from crowds at a pedestrian cross-walk or crossing the road to walk on the pavement with fewer people. One particular aspect of reducing touch and proximity was a change to the Western greeting practice of shaking hands. According to Philippa McGuinness (2021), handshakes have long 'existed within the uneasy space humans negotiate between our desire for touch and our fear of contamination'. The handshake forms not just a common, everyday practice, but is the image of iconic moments of greeting, agreement, truce, treaty and the demystification of those perceived to be 'other'. Many, of course, already expressed concern about the transmission of viral particles and illness-causing bacteria in a handshake – the hilarious obsession of Vice President Selina Meyer (Julia Louis-Dreyfus) in the North American comedy series *Veep* (2012–19) applying sanitizer after regular handshakes with both strangers and friends was funny because it had become an increasingly common practice in the decade before COVID-19. Nevertheless, to lose that capacity for shaking hands to perform a range of necessary social functions for fear of transmitting or catching a serious disease presents a substantial shift to how we perform our corporeal subjectivity in relation to one another.

Handshakes, of course, are not the only social mechanism of greeting and agreement in the world, and it was notable that some of our practices shifted very quickly to adopt other cultural habits and observances that are safer, reduce the proximity of bodies and avoid touch. Early in the pandemic, substantial media coverage and Twitter debate was given over to footage of the then Prince Charles, Prince of Wales, adopting the Namaste instead. As a greeting, namaste avoids touch, placing hands together over the chest and giving a slight bow – namaste is a Sanskrit term to describing bowing to the other as a customary mark of respect, honour and welcome, familiar across the Indian subcontinent (Maguire 2020). For many, the perceived customs of namaste became a suitable mechanism for respectful greeting where handshakes were not recommended.

Others adopted forms of greeting such as the fist bump (closed fists touching), which was not necessarily perceived as substantially less risky than a handshake, but drew on existing variations on shaking hands, allowing touch between two bodies with a mild reduction in the corporeal vulnerability of putting one's fingers and palms into the hands – literally – of others. Another variation on this was the elbow bump, used by many politicians in Western countries around the world, often with excessive jovial display. Again, safer than shaking hands since unlike hands it is impossible to put one's elbow to the face, nose or mouth. However, it was also seen by many to be problematic given the elbow's proximity to the crook into which people were widely encouraged to sneeze and cough (Centers for Disease Control and Prevention 2022). Significant here, of course, is not the fact of bumping elbows as a form of greeting or agreement, but the way in which the laughter often accompanying it indicated the necessity of humour to cope with a substantial social change.

Humour is not, of course, diametrically opposed to seriousness and credibility (McKee et al. 2018: 4583), but is often deployed to allay a sense of vulnerability or precarity (Turton-Turner 2007: 420), and as a coping strategy for resilience in the face of adversity or uncertainty (McCann et al. 2013: 66), which can include unfamiliar or altered customary practices or habits. Here, humour accompanies the shift from normative, barely conscious practices of hand-shaking to alternatives which remind in a very corporeal capacity of the very substantially changed circumstances of touch. I know I am not alone, myself, in adopting humour or the uncertain laughter when navigating the complex and awkward circumstances of doing something different with the body in relation to others – pulling back from the cheek-kiss with those for whom it has been a normal greeting, being unsure whether or not to hug or pulling away from person choosing to sit on a train carriage nearby because the anxiety over transmission of COVID-19 was beginning to change the ways our bodies unconsciously behave with one another.

Forms of communication that include touch are almost always signifiers of welcome or hospitality, whether that is greeting or agreement. For Derrida (2001), an ethics of welcome or hospitality is not something which is cultivated and does not emerge simply through culture but precedes it by virtue of the formulation that ethics *is* hospitality. To act in a manner of hospitality is not necessarily always an ethical hospitality, 'because being at home with oneself … supposes a reception or inclusion of the other which one seeks to appropriate, control, and master according to different modalities of violence' (17). Hospitality depends on a paradox of ontology: an interruption of the self by the self as other (Derrida 1999: 52). In that respect, hospitality depends on the *interruption* of the subject with itself. In the case of the disrupted or altered practices of *communicating* hospitality through touch, the self is doubly interrupted: not only does one give over the self through an act of touch in the performativity of welcome given in the greeting, but the self that is obliged to *hesitate* and decide on the *form* of signalling hospitality speaks to a substantial re-configuration in a normative practice of ontology in the encounter with another. While the destabilization of these norms draws attention to the interruption of the self, the re-stabilization in alternative forms – namaste, the fist- or elbow-bump, the nod, the at-distance air-kiss, the laughed off wave at moderate proximity – indicates the significance of affirming hospitality, and the drive to do so in ways which manage risk.

Managing touch and how bodies touch each other is in itself a practice of hospitality – not touching people inappropriately, avoiding contact with strangers who pass by, and so on. However, it is often even more complex than that when it comes to illness and communicable disease. For example, from early after the discovery of HIV, those who were living with HIV had bodies that were rendered untouchable (Chapman 2000), so much so that when the Princess of Wales – the late wife of the Prince of Wales mentioned above – visited a unit at Middlesex Hospital, London, and shook the hand of a man with HIV without wearing gloves, it made international news and has been credited with significantly challenging misinformation that HIV could be passed through touch (BBC 2017). Here, practices of care included people with HIV themselves avoiding touching others until the transmissibility was better understood, while others actively touching as an act of care. Similarly and more recently, parts of West Africa affected by Ebola developed practices of social distancing and the avoidance of touch as a formation of care to avoid the risk of infecting others, no matter how small that risk may have been (Brown and Sáez 2021). Here, we see the complex negotiation of practices of care of the self and care of the other coincide with disease and infection, whereby touch becomes not something avoided purely out of fear, but a social function that refigures normative practices of bodily proximity.

Reconfiguring the social body of touch

Why is touch important to identity? A very pedestrian (and problematic) common account suggests that the need for touching and being touched is an essential and biological part of human existence. That may be so, although of course any recourse to biology as an explanation for a cultural practice reads biology, nature and the body as somehow extra-discursive and external to culture. A more useful explanatory framework can emerge when we think about the constitution of subjectivity through the materialization of the body as a vulnerable, corporeal self. From the very beginning of subjectivity or indeed before there even is a subject, the body is made less vulnerable through touch, being held, embraced and cared for in ways that warrant touch. Touch, being touched, being in close proximity to other bodies at the complex, constructed point of the threshold of skin is a foundational, *a priori* condition of survival: we are given over to others in close proximity in order to be cared for (Butler 2003: 19–20), whether that care is experienced 'in feeding or in sleeping or in being touched or held' (Butler 2020: 98). This point emerges from the fact that, as infants, before we have consciousness or subjectivity, we are helpless and dependent on the touch of others, which leads to important questions as to how touch is negotiated across the lifecycle when autonomy, authority over one's own body, the capability to have a choice over how one is touched or with whom one is in close bodily proximity was never fully our own in the constitution and constructedness of our subjectivity (Bell 2010: 137).

This means the bodily proximity to the point of touch has always been a complicated and multiple framework of being and performativity in everyday life, situated in complex negotiations and grey areas of consent, care, desired and unwanted touch, of bodies close enough that they appear to be touching uncomfortably, and of touches, caresses and bumps that communicate little, touches that are familiar and unfamiliar, those that are wanted and those that are abject. As Eve Sedgwick (2003: 14) noted, 'the sense of touch makes nonsense out of any dualistic understanding of agency and passivity'. This means that even as conscious, self-aware and reflective adults we are not always engaged with or in control of how we touch or how others are touched – it is an unassailable fact of living in a spatial setting of interdependency in which we must come into contact with other people.

What happens then when ordinary practices of touch and proximity (the bump, the scratch, the knock, brushing up against another, bodies that are within one metre of one another, and so on) are suddenly re-figured as risky? As a risk to the very survivability of corporeal life that began with the necessity of proximity and touch? It is, of course, the case that initial beliefs that COVID-19's transmission was primarily passed by touch (whereby prevention was by sanitizing hands regularly) were replaced later in 2020 with a clearer understanding that the virus particles were transmitted most easily through aerosolized droplets communicated by close proximity to an infected person (whereby the preventative measures required the introduction of masks). Nevertheless, the concerns around proximity and touch have been an ongoing factor in how we prevent the spread of the virus, resulting in proximity and touch becoming complex factors of everyday life to negotiate in ways different from those negotiations we experienced prior to the pandemic.

People experience and engage with touch and proximity in very diverse ways, of course, as part of that grey area of primary negotiation we all experience. In that context, it would be improper to suggest that touch and proximity themselves became perceived as equally abject, risky or dangerous for all people across the globe. Rather, it is more appropriate to suggest that the public health discourse that required reduced touch and, in many jurisdictions, mandated distance between proximate bodies circulated a discourse in which the 'touchy' topic of touch and corporeal proximity became one which called upon subjects to *consider* the extent to which touch and proximity *might* be abject, even if many disavowed or ignored that call, or engaged with it in their own complex ways across the myriad, diverse bodies we encounter in daily life.

There has been a long and very problematic history in which certain kinds of touch and bodily proximity have been coded as abject in ways which shape social relations and identity. Barely-conscious and affectively-felt experiences of disgust turn often on proximity to bodies, their smells and their touch (Probyn 2000: 131; Cover 2015). Sara Ahmed (2004: 54) points out that the refusal of a white woman, for example, to touch a black child is not merely to withdraw or recoil from that which an individual sees as abject, but actively reforms social space by establishing or reinforcing codes of apartness. These, of course, are all part of the negotiations of touch and proximity based on unethical demarcations between bodies, marking some as untouchable (Appadurai 2004). However, when bodily touch and proximity themselves become framed by a discourse of risk, those demarcations are – theoretically, potentially – levelled out: bodies that would not normally be demarcated as untouchable are now not to be touched, or to be near; bodies that were not culturally positioned as abject are now bodies that we cannot have near us; and bodies that were to be avoided are joined by bodies we desired to touch or be near. In other words, the practices of touchable bodies and proximities that previously gave a sense of subjectivity through a framing of corporeal difference across interdependency are re-configured such that how we produce and perform the self in relation to other bodies is – potentially, theoretically – altered.

Practices of touch and proximity depend, of course, on spatial settings as well as the identities of the subjects involved. There are two specific settings related to the pandemic in which practices of touch were disrupted or refigured in ways which speak to subjectivity and belonging, and both of these occur in the context of medicine and health professional work. As we know from Foucault (1973) proximity and touch between a doctor and a patient are a key institutional and cultural formation of identity practices, positioning bodies into those of the expert and the object. As with many other highly communicable diseases, COVID-19 necessitated a change to the ordinary practice of touch and proximity in medical settings, hospitals and general practitioner clinics. I am sure I was not alone in having a routine medical appointment in which a practitioner was masked, gowned and gloved in a way which puts a conceptual distance between myself and the doctor *because* our bodies are in proximity. Naturally, this is a necessary precaution for all parties, given the increased risk of coming into contact with SARS-CoV-2 in a medical setting. At the same time, however, it shifts the ordinary camaraderie between doctor and patient, presenting both our bodies at risk.

Here, the dual frameworks of hospitality and institutional practice in the setting of the clinic that ordinarily enables (or requires) proximity and touch are re-configured in a way which calls upon the patient to see their body not as diseased, dangerous, risky or abject, but as potentially so. The unwillingness to touch – without disposable gloves, at least – becomes a psychic metaphor for the body that is vulnerable to disease. That, too, has significant ethical implications in that there is value in recognizing one's own vulnerability as a shared capacity of corporeal life, but in times of pandemic precarity, to be *positioned* through non-touch is to be framed as a 'problem body'. Our bodies are, of course, diverse and how we figure them as a material part of subjectivity varies widely. However, in the shared experience of the pandemic with the stark reminders of how our bodies carry and convey disease to others and are at risk of having that disease transmitted to us, we are called upon not just to perceive our bodies as vulnerable, but to practice our engagement with others in a way that is over-determined by the perception of the vulnerability of touch and proximity.

Secondly, there is the question of inter-cultural practices of touch in relation to dying and death. Bodies are materialized from the very beginning of life through practices of care that absolutely require touch and proximity, and there are potential instances across an ordinary lifecycle in which the refusal to touch may be perceived as a violent act because it refuses to provide necessary care (Butler 2020). For example, a refusal to hold a child, an unwillingness to bathe or feed a newborn, a recoiling from washing the elderly or infirm are all acts of violence because they withhold care (The Care Collective 2020). One very significant practice of touch involves touching the dying. In addressing some of the ways in which cross-cultural practices merge at the intersection of corporeality and ethics, Alphonso Lingis (1994) identified the touch of consolation for the unwell and, particularly, the dying as a commonality that crosses practices and languages, that signifies beyond other communicative systems. To be near the dying, to remain in proximity and to touch or hold the person who is dying – even if they are completely unknown to us – is a key expression of human ethics, an acknowledgement of the interdependency that precedes our own subjectivity.

Across much of the world, risk-averse hospitals participating in practices to reduce the likelihood of in-and-out transmission of COVID-19 prevented visitors, which included preventing families from being with those who were seriously unwell and those who were dying (whether COVID-19 or other causes). The desire to be with the dying other in the shock of the pandemic was for many a palpable force, and the denial through regulatory practices was seen as an injury because it prevented the fulfilment of the deeply felt obligation towards the dying. Certainly, this was one of the major complaints about lockdowns, immobility and social distancing in many jurisdictions (Turner and Evans 2020). Some attempts to enable virtual visitation of the dying (through video conference) were made by some institutions, although these were seen as causes of greater stress for the surviving family members and partners when the dying patient was catatonic, having breathing difficulties (common in COVID-19 deaths) or intubated and unable to speak, likewise commonly experienced among the seriously unwell with COVID-19 (Downer and Kekewich 2021). This is where Lingis' point about touch for the dying and the seriously unwell transcends linguistic barriers and thereby serves as a form of communication that is called upon as an ethical engagement between subjects and others. As an act or practice which speaks to a deep-seated, intercultural and post-linguistic ethics, that calls upon attendance upon the dying in a way that is deeply implicated with proximity and touch. That such a significant force in everyday practices of caring for the self through caring for the other (the sick, the dying) via a very corporeal ethical engagement was denied was an affront not merely to family relations and practices of care and love, but to the constitutional framework of subjectivity in belonging. Being *with* the dying (touching, in proximity) is significant because it calls to an originary ethics of interdependency that precedes subjectivity itself (Levinas 1969).

Two things occur, then, in the denial of touch and proximity for the dying. On the one hand, the act of hospitality towards the dying that is engaged through touch and proximity is an act which calls into question the 'I' (Levinas 1969: 171), because the subject is linguistically constituted by its other, which includes not just the otherness of other bodies, but the fact that the living 'I' is constituted by the other 'dying' them. Our being is, in Levinas and Lingis' framework, an existence *for* the other with deeply seated obligations towards the other (Levinas 1969: 261). On the other hand, the denial of visitation to the dying does not solidify the 'I' as a subject of self-interest, putting risk ahead of the need to touch the dying, but re-configures the I away from an obligation towards the dying individual – whether familiar or a stranger – and instead towards the precarity of the population as a whole in a temporal disruption. That is, the other who must be cared for is the corporeal being who, as a result of our touching the dying, will die too because we risk spreading the virus through a chain of transmissions. Protecting the unknown body whose death *may come* as a result of our obligation to the *already dying* presents a splitting of the obligation for the other in which the withdrawal of the ethics conveyed through touch and proximity is figured as the 'greater' obligation.

In what ways, then, is it possible to explain the importance of changed conditions of proximity and touch and how it re-configures subjectivity in the context of altered practices of belonging? Significant in our re-figuration of touch and proximity is not how it makes us *feel*, or how we might *distance ourselves* from the touch of others, but the fact that we are constituted in spatial settings that involve bodies in interdependent movement in which touch and proximity are not merely ordinarily a risk but a formation of belonging that operates very much at a psychic level. Our psychic connection to space is, of course, one which is built on an assemblage between built spaces, infrastructure and the organized and disorganized presence of other bodies in varying degrees of proximity to our own, constructing and constituting ourselves as part of an assemblage of bodies that are in touch with one another (Grosz 1995: 108).

That is, the fact we negotiate a range of practices of touch and bodily proximity is because we are corporeally located in space with others in ways that form an assemblage that, itself, is constitutive of our identities. To unpack a little further how an assemblage works, we can draw on Elizabeth Grosz' understanding of the relationship between the body and the city in which the body moves (the city being a useful metaphor for a space that includes the bodies of others). For Grosz (1995: 105), there are two problematic models of the body and the city. In the first, the city is seen as a *reflection* of the body in which bodies are understood mythically to pre-date the city, and the city is designed around the needs and practices of our bodies, as if those bodies are timeless. This view tends towards a one-way relationship between bodies and cities in which the city is always the *effect* of the needs of the body. To put this perspective into the setting of viral prevention, it would suggest that our spaces and environments have been developed in ways that allow movement of bodies that touch – such as being seated next to a stranger on a train – and that the built space or environment must change in order to accommodate unchanging needs of the body. Indeed, what was discovered since the start of the COVID-19 pandemic was the needs of our bodies *did* indeed change – our bodies required space from one another, our bodies required infrastructure that enabled medical examination without touch and our bodies required capabilities for being with the dying without risking transmission of the virus to others – that is, changes to our corporeal practices for which the infrastructure of our environment was not able to adapt. We changed, not the space in this model.

The second model of bodies and cities to which Grosz objected involves the association of cities and states, whereby the historical city-state had sometimes been described as having been designed on the *basis* of the body, for example, that it has a 'head' (the city's prince or leader), a set of arms (its military) and a body (its people, and buildings) and bowels (its waste infrastructure), veins (its roads and walkways) and so on (105–6). This model is perhaps less applicable than the first to how we think about our post-COVID bodies in the context of touch and networks of care and dependency, although of course the idea of transmission through a population was sometimes made representable through models of the body rather than models of diverse networks. Certainly, the idea that a city, space, region or built environment was bound together the way a body binds cells, and the removal of the infected appendage through creating zones of immobility and borders deployed this modelling of space upon the body.

Grosz' solution to the conceptual ineffectiveness of the two common models of bodies and spaces above has been to view the relationship between the two as neither the first (the human body *causes* the built environment and infrastructure) nor the second (the city or space represents the body) but instead as assemblages of body-space. Again, using the metaphor of the city, Grosz wrote:

> What I am suggesting is a model of the relations between bodies and cities that see them, not as megalithic total entities, but as assemblages or collections of parts, capable of crossing the thresholds between substances to form linkages, machines, provisional and often temporary sub-or micro-groupings. This model is practical, based on the productivity of bodies and cities in defining and establishing each other. It is not a holistic view, one that would stress the unity and integration of city and body, their 'ecological balance'. Rather, their interrelations involve a fundamentally disunified series of systems, a series of disparate flows, energies, events, or entities, bringing together or drawing apart their more or less temporary alignments.
>
> (108)

If we perceive of our relationship with space not as bodies thrown into space where there is proximity and touch with other bodies, but as operating in and constituted *as* an assemblage, linkages, provisional and contingent clusterings that make things happen in disunified interrelationality, then we can see better perhaps how the various mechanisms of touch, closeness, proximity and engagement among bodies are a key component of how we perform subjectivities of belonging.

These disunified and contingent encounters that produce various components in an assemblage are, then, the very cause of vulnerability to disease – clusters of bodies that come together at various times in close proximity (those who work in open plan offices and groups of cubicles; those who travel in a packed train car; those who we touch as our purchase is bagged and handed over to us) that permit transmission as the ever-changing machinery of bodies in space are normative processes of proximity and movement away into proximity with others. It is a constitutive force, such that when a prohibition on touch and proximity through regulations of social distancing comes into play, the entire assemblage has to be re-written. If our subjective belonging is constituted in interrelational assemblage of constant changing proximities, the adjustment of the assemblage presents a rupture in subjectivity itself. More significantly, however, this perspective points to the way in which we are a constitutive assemblage with the virus itself by the originary fact of being bodies in space that, by necessity, touch.

The crowd

In many jurisdictional settings, touch and proximity were not wholly forbidden. Rather, they became regulated such that certain kinds of proximities were permitted. For example, in the UK, a 'support bubble' framework was introduced to allow two households to have 'close contact' with another (UK Department of Health and Social Care 2020). The support bubble concept was highly regulated, making it illegal for anyone to engage in the framework if not eligible. Principally, it served those who would otherwise be alone, single parents or under the age of eighteen living in a group with no adults, and could therefore join a household of any size and maintain close contact with them. While social distancing was expected, it is reasonable to assume that the proximity and touch among that support bubble was enough to transmit COVID-19 without while other households remained locked down.

Significant here is that this is touch and proximity clustered and bubbled outside of the assemblage described in the last section. Indeed, what is most important about this is that it permitted some regulated closeness and touch without that being the casual touch among a crowd where the virus is recognized to transfer to bodies with minimal tracking. The denial of crowds of bodies is, of course, sensible as an ordinary, long-standing mechanism of prevention, quarantine and immobility as described in Chapter 4. However, at the same time, it draws on a much older discourse that positions the crowd as problematic, unruly and dangerous. *Large numbers* of bodies in close proximity are not necessarily bodies that can be regimented or that can permit touch and contact to be easily tracked. Crowds of bodies are seen to be dangerous and in need of management (literally: crowd management) when in a state of entertainment or pleasure (Huizinga 1949: 2), when individual composure and ethical behaviour suffer submergence in the setting of a crowd (Munt 2007: 14), or when a natural catastrophe results in an anguished crowd that represents the 'force of nature' itself (Muecke 2007: 260). This is to understand the crowd of bodies together as the multitude or 'mob' that is disorderly, untrackable and unruly, in need of social regulation (Urry 2007: 8).

Ordinarily, our proximity to (and within) crowds, multitudes and mobs operates across modes of chosen and unchosen, and the unchosen crowd with whom we are part of an assemblage of bodies in space is an unassailable fact of our necessary cohabitation of space (Butler 2015: 27). The regulation of touch and proximity by forms of quarantine and immobility, prevention of visiting, distanced medical appointments and the wholesale prevention of crowds shifts the bounds of cohabitation with bodies in space. Here, the normally crowded streets are not only made empty by the prevention of crowds; rather, we suffer the loss of our engagement with the disorderly multitude as an everyday practice of identity that confirms our belonging to populations (Cover 2020a) while also making us vulnerable to disease through the *unruly casualness* of proximity and touch.

Performativity incorporates not merely the patterns and pathways through which we construct, as a process, our sense of identity over time in ways which are stabilized and normative. Rather, part of the performativity of identity involves the randomness of the casual touch, the bodies that are brought into proximity with others – including particularly strangers – and the corporeal unknowability of what will happen as we move through, within and along with a crowd. It is part of the recognition that we cohabit a world, that this cohabitation precedes and thereby constitutes us and that cohabitation of space with strangers and familiars is beyond our agency. While preventing the crowd as a means of slowing down the transmission of the virus through reducing the flows of bodies that come into proximity, touch and enable the mobility of disease is a powerful tool to save lives of those with whom we cohabit that we do not know and may never meet, its absence from everyday life is reconstitutive of the subjects formed by encounter with that crowd.

Staying in touch

Touch, of course, is part of a practice of connection with others (Probyn 2005: 10), but it is not and never has been the *only* practice in which we connect, perform belonging, communicate affection or fulfil needs related to our being socially constituted as social subjects. Putting aside the somewhat complex concerns of not being able to touch, be near or communicate with the dying due to social distancing and quarantine frameworks, and the failure of alternatives such as video-conferencing to perform those actions (Downer and Kekewich 2021), it remains that social connection or what we often call colloquially 'staying in touch' does not require the physical proximity and closeness of bodies that was often demanded as necessary for mental health and well-being during the social distancing and physical separations of the pandemic safety measures.

Arguably, our very cultural practices of technological development have been framed by a deep-seated desire or demand for the capability to communicate and connect with others without the need for touch or proximity. Popular and pedestrian technological determinist models of communication tools often describe the social changes of technologies as if those technologies were an accident of invention that brought both positive and negative changes on how we behave. Cultural theorist Raymond Williams (1990: 10–11) was critical of technological determinist theories that viewed the invention of a technology as an accident or an individual invention, unrelated to existing needs, desires and demands, that then goes on to have an impact on society, change institutions and practices, and produce other unforeseen consequences. He offered an approach that sought to restore *intention* to the understanding of technological development, such that new technologies are not seen as an accident or the work of an individual 'inventor' who discovers a technology that subsequently causes widespread social change, but as 'actively looked for and developed with certain purposes in mind' including 'known social needs, purposes and practices to which the technology is not marginal but central' (13). Using the example of television, Williams pointed out that contrary to popular myths, there is no singular event or moment of television's invention – rather, there was a process of development, investment, trial and construction over half a century to produce a technology which responded to a cultural demand or desire to bring moving images into the domestic setting of the private home.

In the same way, other media and communication technologies that enable us to 'stay in touch' with others through real-time and recorded conversation – the telephone, the text message, email, video-conferencing – are all responses to a cultural desire or demand for social connection and communication across vast spaces without the need for the kinds of proximities and corporeal closeness that was once required for real-time communication (or for which letters delivered provided a slow-form recorded option). Rather than figuring the social distancing practices of pandemic health measures as creating a 'lack' of touch, there may be value in recognizing that it while it constituted a breach in everyday practice of corporeal proximity and engagement for many with crowds, it was much less an absence and more across a shift from one deeply desired form of social connection (enabled by mobility and closeness) towards another deeply desired cultural practice of social connection (enabled by communication technologies).

Finally, it is worth remarking that while subjective and performative practices of intimacy often involve touch, it is always an over-simplification to assume they *must* involve touch and corporeal proximity. As Sedgwick (2003: 17) has noted, this idea is already betrayed by the use of the word 'touching' to describe feeling without the necessity of tactility, much as the 'staying in touch' described above deploys a term that makes tactility the 'gold standard' of connectivity while simultaneously suggesting that it is always constituted in its range of alternatives. In other words, connection occurs in many other ways, including forms that do not rely on the communication technologies mentioned above. That is, forms of intimacy, entanglement and reciprocity can operate through other senses that do not depend on proximity of skin to skin (Probyn 2005).

Rather, intimacy, interest and connection can be – and often are – performed through other corporeal practices of engagement such as visuality and looking (Lingis 1994: 173), whereby bodies that are in sight of each other can practice connectivities across a room, across a street, through a window, through protective barriers designed to prevent the exchange of air and aerosolized viral practices, and so on. In the same way the aural experience of hearing the voice of a familiar person through a closed door protecting oneself from infection can be an act of connection that need not be measured against touch as the marker of intimacy but operate merely as an alternative intimate engagement. This was undoubtedly the experience of many households in which one member was infected with COVID-19 while others remained safe but audible, intimately connected (and not abandoning their intimates) with neither sight nor touch nor the familiarity of smell. Significant here is that there are a range of practices of engagement, connection and intimacy between people, and while the requirements of social distancing adjusted the formation of touch as a marker of connection and cohabitation with others in the world, it did not necessarily eradicate intimacy and connection. Indeed, it could be argued that foregrounding alternative forms of connection that do not rely on touch and corporeal proximity can be factors fostering resilience among those who generated a sense of disconnection resulting from the necessary distance between bodies.

Conclusion

Touch and the close proximity of bodies are, as I have been describing it, a highly significant element in the performativity of our selfhood as subjects of belonging and cohabitation of space. There are certainly cultural practices and discourses that establish norms of touch and proximity, although these norms are regularly debated, miscommunicated, negotiated and formations of both anxiety and pleasure. In an era marked by the desire not to misinterpret intentions of touch – such as in ensuring the connectivity's clarity of difference between the touch that supports, the corporeal proximity of friendship or necessity and the nearness that is a flirtation (Bartlett et al. 2019), the very idea of bodies that are in proximity or 'touching distance' is made more complex and more guarded. In that sense, touch and bodily proximity are always about vulnerability, but how that vulnerability is experienced is *both* a shared condition of being corporeal *and* diversely experienced across those multiple negotiations that are necessary in an everyday space cohabited with other people.

The social distancing measures adopted, recommended or mandated in many jurisdictions around the world presented a new framework in which touch and close proximity of bodies became not forbidden but further complicated: shifting how we perform greetings and agreement, how we perform intimacy, how care professionals who rely on touch to perform their roles do so, how we practice our rituals of proximity to the dying and how we move about in ever-changing crowds of bodies. The fact that our culturally desired technologies of communication have long enabled connection without touch became a key aspect in the performance of belonging for many, whether those of us forcibly locked down in immobility and separation, or those who self-regulated to protect from transmission. Touch and close proximity, therefore, became a matter of identity performance subject not only to norms and negotiations, but to regulatory practices and ethical obligations to *not* risk transmission through close proximity. With the pandemic continuing – although normalized in some respects now in everyday life in many parts of the world – it is too soon to know if our practices of touch and proximity are broadly changed conceptually or practically, or if other changes and cautionary measures that prevent touch and proximity from becoming acts of violence have been furthered by the recognition that corporeal life is a life marked by vulnerabilities and pleasures in bodily closeness.

7

Disrupted corporealities: Vaccination and anti-vaxxers

Introduction

The development of a vaccine that would reduce the serious effects of COVID-19 infection, including its mortality, and lessen the risk of transmission of the virus, was a serious game-changer over the pandemic years. While the development and availability of vaccines and the roll-out of vaccination to more than half of the world's population (unevenly, of course) in no way 'ends' the pandemic, it substantially altered the framework of health regulations and the wholesale dependence on immobility, lockdowns and social distancing as mandatory, encouraged or desirable practices for the survival of life. Many of us might reasonably have assumed from the start that the development and roll-out of a vaccine programme would be celebrated as an indication of the strengths of international scientific knowledge frameworks, of the genuine possibilities of human civilization to respond to major global issues or – perhaps somewhat problematically – as an opportunity to draw on Enlightenment patriarchal thinking and see the vaccine as evidence of human 'domination' and 'mastery' of something considered 'nature'. And, of course, as heralding the possibilities that the necessary health restrictions would end. However, the force and spread of anti-vaccination discourses, disinformation, hostility, protest and violence over vaccine mandates in many jurisdictions and, even more worryingly, over the vaccine itself was genuinely surprising.

A small but growing anti-vaccination lobby has existed for many years, particularly in the United States, Europe and Australia (Brennan 2018). However a new anti-COVID vaccination and anti-mandatory vaccination movement was built around the convergence of those anti-vaxxer discourses and an anti-establishment populist framework of institutional distrust and individualism. For the most part, in many Western countries, this anti-vaccination movement was very vocal but ultimately very small, and did not actually prevent the majority from taking up vaccination once available. Of greater importance was the less-vocal vaccine hesitancy that either delayed people from becoming vaccinated or drove them towards anti-vaccination attitudes.

A great deal has already been written about the social setting of COVID-19 vaccination, the role of disinformation and conspiracy theory in creating difficulties for the roll-out of vaccination programmes, how vaccine hesitancy works, the infiltration of alt-right populists into an existing anti-vaxxer movement, the violence of protests against vaccine mandates and family breakdowns resulting from divergent opinions on vaccination. Although all of these have very important implications for identity, belonging and sociality in the COVID years, there is no need to rehearse all of that insightful work here in detail. Rather, what I would like to do in this chapter is address one core aspect of the intersection of COVID vaccination debates and identity: the perception of risk and how a concept of risk draws on the ways in which identities have been positioned over the past century while serving also as a performative act of both selfhood and fragmented social affiliation. At stake in the understanding of risk is the juxtaposition and difficulty of recognizing and apprehending risk in terms of both population health (risk to others if remaining unvaccinated) and individual bodies (perceived risk of vaccination). Here perhaps is where we see the pivoting between interdependency and individualism at its greatest during the pandemic, whereby global populations are called upon to position themselves within that complex arrangement of subjectivity in ways which have become difficult in an era of hostile politics and rampant faith in the figure (and assumed 'rights') of the individual. To work through this, I will begin with a brief positioning of vaccination and vaccine mandates and how they operate in terms of the cultural concept of 'population' rather than individualized or transactional health, before addressing how the anti-vaccination anxiety and vaccine hesitancy was produced as a cultural formation. This will be followed by a discussion of risk and calculation as a form of identity performativity before ending the chapter with a further discussion of how the differences between individual risk management and social risk conscious of interdependency call upon a new ethical perspective for how we calculate risk for ourselves and others.

Important here is not to assume questions of vaccination, failing to be vaccinated or being vaccine-hesitant are personal choices made exclusively through a practice of agency. This would be to romanticize the individual subject of agency which, as we know from decades of poststructuralist intervention

(Butler and Spivak 2007: 41), is to divorce subjectivity from the trace of the discourses, cultural practices and assumptions that actively constitute us, and the fact that no choice or decision can ever be made separate from the working of contemporary power, language and sociality. In other words, it is easy – or lazy – to slam those who were hesitant about or outrightly refused vaccination as ignorant, selfish or inappropriately adversarial, but when considered from cultural and ethical perspectives it is important to recognize that the responsibility for those decisions (if they ever were fully decisions) does not rest exclusively with individuals but the cultural formations that produce them.

The vaccine story

Vaccines have been around for two centuries and are very much a tried-and-tested health measure in response to communicable viruses. For those many people who do not work in the health sciences or professions, a lot of learning about vaccination was done during 2021 and 2022, with regular news stories, explainers, documentaries and other circulated knowledge about vaccines, how they work and how new practices such as mRNA vaccine technologies developed. We learned, for example, that vaccination developed in response to smallpox in the late eighteenth century, although there had been earlier knowledges in China and elsewhere that introduced smallpox scab material to uninfected individuals as a nasal powder as an early form of inoculation (Silverstein 2009). British physician Edward Jenner, we learned, developed the smallpox vaccine using the virus that caused the much milder cowpox – and that our everyday term vaccination is derived from the Latin word *vaccinus* ('from the cow'). Although much of the media and public sphere discourse was on the emergent COVID-19 vaccinations, a resurgence in stories about other vaccines circulated so that a wider public gained new knowledge that rightly positioned vaccination as one of the most efficient mechanisms for preventing both mortality from viruses and the spread of viruses, and in some cases coming close to the eradication of serious communicable viruses (Centers for Disease Control and Prevention 2011). In other words, COVID-19 was the cause in many parts of the world for a renewed history lesson of human and scientific intervention in disease management and prevention.

Significant in the history of vaccination is that this very successful technique pre-dates by nearly a century the scientifization of antibiotics which have formed our 'go to' response to bacterial and other infections for much of the twentieth century. Vaccination pre-dates the important work of Louis Pasteur in the development of microbial germ theory, the elimination of pathogens in milk and other animal produce through heat ('pasteurization') and the most substantial development in attenuating or weakening a microbe's virulence in order to produce effective and safe vaccines. For Foucault (2007: 57–9), the fact that vaccination pre-dates the scientific developments over the following century that allowed them to be understood in rational, scientific terms is part of the developing framework of 'securitizing' the population, going hand-in-hand with shifts in power frameworks that encourage institutions and governance mechanisms to apply pastoral care to the wider population to encourage life and liveability. Across this historical path, for many in Western countries and other regions, vaccination became an *ordinary* part of the practice of *belonging* to a wider population (Cover 2020a), whereby that belonging is performed through various ritualistic acts such as the automatic and unquestioned vaccination of children. In other words, in everyday life vaccination is so routine and unremarkable it has been 'un-thought' because there is nothing particularly remarkable about it.

Part of what is 'un-thought' that makes vaccination drop into the background of everyday life has been the mandatory requirement for certain vaccines in some jurisdictions and the practice of administrative record-keeping by state agencies to monitor vaccine programmes. Indeed, as early as the first decade of the nineteenth century vaccine mandates began to appear in Europe. In 1806, Elisa – sister to Napoleon Bonaparte who was given by him the rule of the Italian principality of Piombino and the republic of Lucca – introduced the first obligatory vaccination programme for smallpox, despite weak support for the new practice of vaccination in other parts of Europe. Elisa required that all adults and infants within two months of birth must be vaccinated (Grab 2015). In light of the growing connection between state governance and public health, disease was understood as a threat to the security of the state and public order, and the response was to draw on rationalist approaches to healthcare and emerging innovations of the medical sciences by mandating vaccination against smallpox. The personnel, policies and practices were resourced and put in place to manage the programme, and adopted elsewhere in Napoleonic Europe (Vigni 2001), and the success of the programme resulted in an increasing awareness of the importance of mandatory, encompassing vaccination programmes by demonstrating the substantial differences in security, health and well-being between jurisdictions that mandated vaccination and those that did not (Lewis 2022b: 79).

Most importantly, however, the continued roll-out of vaccination as a normative feature of governance throughout many parts of the world operated at the intersection between disciplinary and biopolitical forms of power, both acting in concert to normalize – with some variance – through regulation, measurement and administrative record-keeping (Foucault 2004a: 242, Foucault 2007: 63). Through the normativization of vaccination, those who do not vaccinate are positioned as abnormal in disciplinary terms and as at a (possibly unacceptable) distance from the norm in a distributional curve in biopolitical terms; the combination of abnormality and non-proximity to a regulatory norm risks making a subject unrecognizable *as* a subject (Foucault 2004b: 292). While the regulatory practice of normativization can often be violent against those who are positioned to fail to perform within a norm's allowable constraints (Butler 1993: 53), the significance of normativization as a discursive practice is not only that it regulates what is to be understood as both 'ordinary' and 'compulsory' for full subjectivity, but it disappears into the backdrop as a cultural formation that can only be highlighted and recognized through critique or contestation. In other words, vaccination became by the late twentieth century a practice so normative that while we might feel inconvenienced by its necessity, and children might cry at the sight of the syringe, and we might suffer some minor ill-effects for a day or two in annoyance, we were not positioned to ask why vaccination is important or to understand its importance as a matter of population health rather than individual need.

The anti-vaxxer anxiety

Given the normativization of vaccination, which I have described above as a cultural practice in many parts of the world, it is somewhat surprising therefore that vocal and violent opposition to vaccines, vaccination programmes and mandatory vaccination regulations emerged so quickly. While there has been much press, public and political speculation as to the cause (disinformation, populism, belligerence and stupidity being the usual targets), when we look at it from a cultural perspective it is important to recognize that there is no one singular cause to the emergence of a cultural formation, including one which defies logic. Rather, it is important to look for some of the historical, discursive and cultural frameworks that converge at this particular time and in the context of a major, global health crisis to understand how vaccine hesitance and vaccine refusal emerged during the pandemic and did so in ways which were sometimes disruptive to the roll-out.

One strand of anti-vaccination anxiety emerged decades before COVID-19 – the anti-vaxxer movement of the late 1990s. Much of the anti-vaxxer thinking was based on an idea that vaccines were harmful to children and relied on a now thoroughly debunked study from 1998 by Andrew Wakefield that made a tentative connection between the Measles, Mumps and Rubella (MMR) vaccine and autism. The article was later proven to be based not only on misreporting of data but fraud, and caused a widespread panic that reduced vaccination rates of children in many parts of the world to well below the 95 per cent needed for herd immunity (Godlee, Smith and Marcovitch 2011). Naturally, as with many conspiracy theories, those who built an identity practice based on that research continue to believe in it, or believe that its discrediting was surreptitiously supporting other agendas.

Aspects of the anti-vaccination movement built at this time became part of the COVID-19 anti-vaxxer movement, providing a core set of resources that disavowed scientific intervention in favour of inaccurate assumptions about natural immunity (Lewis 2022b: 67) or problematic collusion between jurisdictional approval authorities and major pharmaceutical companies (Anselmi 2018: 80–1). The rhetoric of the extant anti-vaxxer movement was key to the development of vaccine hesitancy and refusal in the context of COVID-19, although this was arguably not the cause (Attwell, Hannah and Leask 2022). Some of the factors that are discernibly new to COVID-19 vaccine refusal and hesitancy – and pertinent to considering vaccination in the context of identity, belonging and risk – include (i) the rise of new forms of disinformation in the years just prior to the pandemic, (ii) increasing populist distrust in institutions and governments, (iii) the communitarianism that formed among a global network of anti-COVID vaccines and (iv) the failure of a wider population, governments and scholars to recognize that the opposition to vaccination was caused by more than just ignorance or a lack of knowledge. I would like to address each of these four briefly in turn.

Disinformation – also sometimes referred to as 'fake news' – is an emergent cultural formation that, from the mid-2010s, became widely used in everyday public discourse to describe a range of problematic texts, content, forms and behaviour, including those that shared deliberately misleading or biased information and propaganda (i.e. disinformation), that that unintentional shared misleading or false information (i.e. misinformation) and other forms fabricated content sometimes mimicking news or factual material (Cover, Haw and Thompson 2022). Although there is a long history of misleading content in the form of propaganda and media bias (Jackall 1995, Freelon and Wells 2020), disinformation operates as a new phase in misleading media content in three respects: (i) its association with interactive, digital platforms which operate without the same strength and extensiveness of editorial gate-keeping familiar in the print and broadcast era; (ii) the widespread public concerns that emerged since 2016 across opinion and news reports, particularly in relation to electoral politics and health communication; and (iii) the way in which disinformation has been positioned as an 'alien' formation warranting technical solutionism, rather than perceived as a cultural emergence that is produced in the very practices of creativity, interactivity and user engagement that it is often perceived as disrupting.

The term disinformation has certainly extended in relation to claims that COVID-19 is a hoax and that vaccination programmes have a hidden agenda (Harvey 2021); it has also been deployed as a term of abuse for those who have advocated a stronger investigation into the origin of the virus, arguably reducing the efficacy of any public communication on investigation and examination that assesses the full range of possible causes (Knott 2021b).

One of the problems of the public perception of disinformation and fake news is the assumption that it is consumed and shared in the context of echo chambers and filter bubbles that, resulting from unfortunate choices, allow platform algorithms to dominate a user's feed with the 'wrong' sort of information or an overload of misleading content. Certainly, echo chambers were often popularly 'blamed' for the production of anti-vaccination sentiment among populations who had not previously been part of earlier anti-vaxxer movements (Kokkegård 2022). Axel Bruns (2019), however, has powerfully demonstrated that exposure to a *range* of discourses as opposed to the singularity found in an echo chamber is far more widespread than often recognized among those who see echo chambers and filter bubbles as the cause of user belief in disinformation. Rather, platform recommendation systems that utilize algorithms may reinforce beliefs or provide evidence for beliefs that have been generated through a more complex cultural engagement (50). However, those who are closely tied to a misleading discourse are, as research has found, often very much engaged in seeking out texts the rest of us regard as credible and verifiable for the purpose of finding material to argue against (Bruns 2019; Cover, Haw and Thompson 2022). So we cannot be as simplistic as blaming online news feeds or echo chambers for people not being exposed to the 'correct' information on the benefits of being vaccinated or the reasons behind the mandatory requirements where they were instituted.

Secondly, being predisposed to distrust statements that put faith in scientific assessment is a more widespread problem, as seen in recent decades in relation to climate science, distrust of 5G networks and other formations of technology. Distrust of vaccines ranged from general uncertainty that there would be no prolonged or damaging side effects to beliefs that mRNA vaccine technology could 're-write human DNA' or that the syringes contained microchips that, once inserted in the body, would allow governments (or Microsoft founder Bill Gates) to track our movements (Lee 2021). The full range of these untrusting attitudes builds on a wider distrust of medical science which, for Foucault (1973: 146), was always understandable since the figure of the medical practitioner was never able to fully synthesize into their practice the persistent spectre of death as both threat and reality – always capable when it is thought to lend suspicion to the practice of medicine. More significantly, of course, a distrust of institutions due to the power differential between professionals and lay-persons has always had the capacity to generate distrust among the general population (Christie and Mittler 1999: 238), and distrust is heightened when the expertise or knowledge to understand aspects of professional and scientific decision-making is low. Certainly, this is the case during the COVID-19 vaccination programmes which saw the first ever use of an mRNA vaccine. Again, this points to the need to avoid the assumption that vaccine refusal or hesitancy was based on a lack of knowledge or understanding and, instead, to look to some of the underlying social and cultural factors that engender distrust, including the rise of a populism that disavows all trust in established institutions.

Claims that personal sovereignty or integrity was threatened by either voluntary or mandatory vaccination programmes was, of course, mythical and served to build populist movements by appealing to the uncertainty and utilizing discourses of risk, vulnerability and alarmism to generate and sustain anger, outrage and dissent in the form recognized among contemporary alt-right populisms (Inglehart and Morris 2016). All populist movements depend on the establishment of adversity through creating a sceptical position of distrust in political institutions and arguing that in mainstream media publications that support them are being partisan or themselves untrustworthy (Daddow 2013). Distrust, on the other hand, deepens societal divisions (Lewis and Weigert 1985), and in this respect COVID vaccine refusal was not merely *about* vaccination but arguably as much a cultural formation in support of populist movements.

Thirdly, there is the question of how a sense of affiliation with others who are hesitant about – or violently opposed to – vaccination operates as a form of *communitarianism*. That is, a sense of community, friendship and bonds of affiliation forms among those who encounter others who find that sense of affiliation among the refusers and hesitant and join their cause. This was certainly the case among the protest culture that formed in opposition to COVID-19 vaccine mandates in Canada and Australia which have been described as 'part festival, part rabble-rousing cry for change' (Lewis 2022b: 27). Significant, of course, is the way in which a festival-style demonstration builds and sustains ties by drawing on aspects of the carnivalesque (Bakhtin 1984). Such a sense of bonded community among those who might otherwise be disconnected from sociality has been witnessed in polarized online abuse and bullying (Cover 2022), and in relation to the spread of conspiracy theories (Lewis 2022b: 34). In both cases, the sense of community, engagement and belonging is recognized as a factor driving adherents into greater devotion to an attitude or disposition to an object of thought over time, with a need to repeat, share and demonstrate faithfulness to that attitude to maintain the network of peers, friends and socialities forged through that adherence.

This, of course, does not just apply to networks of belonging developed by direct participation in demonstrations and protests, but those whose adherence to anti-vaccination sentiment is forged through consumption and sharing of the discourses of disavowal. Audiences, digital users and those who consume, engage with and interactively share texts that belong to a marginal or alternative discourse forge a 'mutual link to a common readership [that] creates a kind of community to which they see themselves as belonging' (Wenger 1998: 182), and this applies regardless of whether or not that engagement involves an online or face-to-face conversation with others in that community. By gaining that sense of affiliation, a subject is positioned to recognize an affective mutuality or affiliation through the shared attitude or utterance, citing the disinformation or statement of opposition to vaccination, and repeating it such that it constitutes a node of performative identity in belonging to what is perceived as community. It is, of course, no surprise that those whose identities might be on the margins of sociality and normative belonging, those who feel disenfranchised or disconnected from what they perceive as the wider sociality and those with inequitable access to the resources necessary for a liveable life are attracted to forms of belonging in adversity, because – at least – it is an opportunity to belong to something. Here, recognizing the power of a sense of belonging is significant in understanding anti-vaccination attitudes: for some, it may not be about the vaccination (at all) but about the sense of engagement and belonging that is forged by that felt experience of affiliation, similitude and symbolic community – sustaining that, of course, warrants hardening attitudes.

Finally, there is the question of ignorance. In many respects, such conspiracy theories and populist outrage is a collapse in the value of trust that stems from the recognition of what Kelly Cole (2004: 95) described as symbolic differences between the exalted and the base – the expert medical scientist or authority and the profit-oriented liar who descends from the snake oil merchant. COVID-19 vaccination is a difficult and complex topic, partly because the science of vaccination is not in itself simple, virology is a complicated 'expert' science and several of the new vaccines utilized new mechanisms such as mRNA technology that, to fully appreciate, require a good understanding of basic genetics and biotechnology. In that sense, a form of non-knowing or inequitable access to knowledge frameworks is obviously at play. However, we need to be very careful not to bash people for a lack of understanding or their minimal resources to forge a framework that can make sense of complex scientific topics. That is, if some people disavow vaccination because – to them – mRNA or other aspects of the vaccines is incomprehensible, it is not necessarily an incomprehensibility for which they are fully responsible.

Part of the confusion over vaccination was the initial presumption that COVID-19 vaccines will produce immunity to infection or re-infection (Lewis 2022b: 100). That, of course, was not the case, with acquired immunity now recognized to wane over time, and early vaccines that failed to prevent the spread of the Omicron variant. The benefit of vaccination is therefore balanced towards reduced – but not prevented – transmissibility and reduced mortality after infection, with some mathematical modelling indicating more than 14 million lives saved during the first year of vaccination (Watson et al. 2022). However, the discrepancy between early understandings of what vaccines *should do* (immunize) and the realisation of their longer-term imperfect effectiveness provided an opportunity for the anti-vaccination lobby and influencers to develop even greater distrust by creating confusing that looked like ignorance among their followers and adherents.

Other misunderstandings, however, hark back to some of the more problematic conspiracy theories about the mRNA vaccines, including the idea that mRNA will alter or 're-write' human DNA or integrate into the human genome, mutating our bodies into something other (Linderman 2021). This, too, builds on older popular discourses that fear genetic and genomic science as something which will modify human identity, producing what Mary Shelley (1992) articulated in her 1818 novel *Frankenstein* as the non-human 'race of devils' – a strand of which has continued through popular entertainment whereby our attachment to human subjectivity and anxieties over its security are played out in horror, fantasy and science fiction texts about the DNA manipulation creating monsters (Cover 2020a: 140). The idea that mRNA vaccines might change human DNA or cause our bodies to 'mutate' (in the popular science fiction sense, not the actual evolutionary sense of mutation) is based entirely on a lack of understanding as to how mRNA vaccines work – they do not enter the cell nucleus where our DNA is found, and the RNA is broken down by cells once it begins to produce the necessary protein (Carballo-Carbajal 2021).

A lack of critical engagement with the science of vaccination is, then, not a surprising cause in some people's trust in the more simplistic disinformation, anti-vaxxer engendering of doubt, or the 'safety' felt among communities of doubters and anti-vaccination protesters. Significant here, however, is *not* to make people responsible for their own ignorance or lack of resources to enable understanding. Ignorance is not a 'lack of knowledge', although we often speak of ignorance in this way, assuming that a person who might be labelled ignorant has simply not read up on a topic, or encountered and learned some important piece of information or routine way of living but with feeding them the correct information that lack or absence can be filled up with understanding (Lewis 2022b: 28). Ignorance, rather, is something that is 'actively produced and maintained' by cultural forces, power arrangements and disciplinary techniques that utilize ignorance as a form of disenfranchisement (Gilson 2011: 309). In that sense, there is limited utility in assuming that a remedy to anti-vaccination and vaccine hesitancy is to be found in better knowledge, more frequent information, less disinformation or better forms of social connectivity. Rather, this is a matter of more ethical *listening* to the hesitant and the disavowers, and understanding the conditions that position a subject to be non-understanding of the science or to place trust in institutional expertise when that understanding is, by the nature of the topic, beyond everyday non-expert knowledge frameworks. I will return to this point in the conclusion of this chapter. In the next section, however, I want to consider one of the core conditions that underlie the capacity of disinformation, populist anti-institutional distrust and communitarianism – the ways in which contemporary subjects have been positioned to address and take on-board 'risk'.

Risk discourses, choices and calculation

Many in public sphere discourse have taken a dichotomous approach to the vaccine refusal and established a set of binaries in which those who are vaccinated are seen as ethical, moral, considerate of their own health and the health of others, versus those who are opposed to vaccination as misled, selfish, disengaged or violent. To do so is not only to leave aside the important fact of vaccine hesitancy among a wider group of people or to improperly misread and stereotype all those opposed to vaccination, but misses the point about how the identity, sociality and belonging operate in the context of the *calculation* of risk. I would like to consider here how we are culturally positioned in the twenty-first century to address risk and to calculate risk as a performative act of subjectivity, and how that plays into a diversity of approaches to the vaccine as something which – rightly – is perceived as entailing risk.

The idea that we live in a 'risk society' was a concept which gained substantial currency in the 1990s, with scholars arguing that shifts away from traditional practices towards a modernity in which society are overwhelmingly driven by a reflexive desire to manage risk individually (Beck 1998). For researchers following the risk society approach, there is seen to be a chronic sensitivity to risk that calls upon agents to manage their own risk – often transactionally – rather than rely on social forms of governance or peer and familial networks for support (Horlick-Jones 2005: 294). While apprehending the role of risk as a factor in how we undertake and perform sociality has value, the theory is sometimes criticized for attempting to define the governing principles of contemporary society by a singular, monolithic concept (Faist 2013: 1639), and for failing to recognize this formation's development in longer, more complex and more diverse process of the securitization of populations described by Foucault (2007). More valuable, here, is to see how risk as a practice of calculation is heightened in particular times of crisis in ways which operate at the interface between the individualized subject and the governance, sociality and practices of belonging to a population.

In the context of population health, for example, risk is a framing factor that governs how we think about and react to disease. Communicable disease has a long history of being understood as a formation assessed and analysed through a discourse of risk that was formulated in the institutionalization of medicine in the seventeenth and eighteenth centuries (Foucault 2007: 60–1). The risk of catching a disease, of dying from it, the beneficial risk taken in being inoculated, the differential risks of mobility and mortality that are specific to different age groups, the risks of not intervening and the risks or benefits of letting a disease spread to create herd immunity are very old frameworks that govern how we think about and understand disease, including today COVID-19. What is important, however, is that a risk focus is not simply a strategy deployed in the context of a high-profile catastrophe or threat such as a pandemic, but a *practice* that comes to infuse everyday life through the deployment of resources to judge, consider, assess and – most importantly – *calculate* strategies in everyday contexts in order to maintain order, predictability and stability (Schehr 2005: 47, Lazzarato 2011: 102).

Part of the practice of neoliberalism is to oblige everyday subjects to participate in the management of risk as an individual rather than socially supported formation. This practice emerged historically in earlier forms of liberalism in which subjects are deliberately stimulated through disciplinary and biopolitical regulation to experience everyday life as a matter of risk, including particularly danger (Foucault 2008: 66). As liberalism re-shaped into neoliberal frameworks in which every aspect of selfhood and sociality became subject to a discourse of economic exchange, wider society became less involved in guaranteeing individuals against risk (whether individually or collectively experienced). Rather, neoliberal regimes call upon subjects to manage that risk based on their own resources (Foucault 2008: 145). This is broadly experienced today as the purchase of insurance against risk, including risks which are normally experienced individually (e.g. corporeal health or the protection of belongings against theft) and those which are experienced collectively (e.g. floods, fire and other catastrophic events that affect whole neighbourhoods, towns or regions), as well as a range of activities to protect against other kinds of risks (e.g. maintaining savings, investing in secure bonds, and so on to protect against economic downturns, job losses, etc.). This creates a biopolitical impetus to be *attentive* to risk as a way of framing our engagement with everyday life, space, other people, institutions and governments in order to participate as a normative subject in contemporary society.

However, the management of risk is more than just a practice of preparing for the possibility of a threat to health, well-being or financial stability. It creates a link between political governance that produces and shares *risk factors* through statistical assessment of whole populations that simultaneously 'massifies' the idea of risks as shared among many and 'individualizes' the concept by seizing upon the body as the object of risk (Clough 2008: 18). Effectively, then, normativity and social participation are built upon a particular framing of risk that places the individual at the centre of the *meaning* of risk. We are trained, disciplined and regimented in risk management as part of engaging socially such that we perform ourselves in relation to others through what Clifton Evers (2008: 423) has identified as personal safety strategies that minimize risk through a process of self-regulation.

Because risk has increasingly been framed as an individualized function of normative belonging, when governments step in to manage risk at the level of the population (as was the necessary case across the health measures in response to COVID-19, including the vaccination programmes), suspicion emerges. This is obviously particularly the case when aspects of that management involve regulatory practices such as lockdowns, social distancing and the mandatory requirement to be vaccinated in order to work or socialize. It is notable that while the routine vaccination of children as I have described it above fell into the *ordinariness* of social participation such that for many years it was unthinkable not to vaccinate a child or consider it as risky, two of our other routine practices of vaccination place the activity at the discretion of the individual: inoculations for travel to places that may put one at risk, and annual influenza vaccines which are optionally taken up by many after encouragement, but rarely if ever mandated. Here, one is called upon to consider the risks through knowledge that is available: will I catch cholera if I am not vaccinated? Will I risk the time away from work if I have some minor side effects from an influenza vaccine or shall I risk the possibility of catching influenza this season? Could that cholera or influenza kill me? How do I weigh up the risk and the cost of the vaccine?

The juxtaposition, then, between a biopolitical administration that mandates vaccines as a strategy against risk (to the population) and the more usual experience of risk whereby the individualized subject decides on matters of health and wellbeing (for their own body) establishes an aporia in which the calculation of risk turns back against governance. Why, after so many years in which risk was moved into the purview of the individual, does governance on behalf of society engage in risk on matters of health? What does it mean to manage the risk to the population, the economy, the well-being of the state by distributing, encouraging or mandating vaccines to protect against risk when the decision to take a risk or understand something as risky has been individualized for so long? What other agenda might there be if governments seem to be suddenly re-entering the field of health risk so ostensibly for the first time in a long time? Can what we are being told about the safety of the vaccines be trusted by a government that does not routinely advise on health risks? These are the questions that ground some aspects of COVID-19 vaccine hesitancy and vaccine refusal, and they are questions that are produced in the context of how risk has been culturally produced in alignment with practices of individuation and selfhood.

They are not, of course, good or sensible or insightful questions – governments all over the world engage in risk management persistently whether in terms of threats to the population (criminal sentencing laws for serial killers, for example, or regulation of car manufacturing and road safety rules to minimize traffic-related injuries), intervening in economic downturns and providing at least some welfare (without which, for example, greater numbers of people will be made homeless or will starve) or determining the risk of health measures (the assessment of pharmaceuticals, vaccines, immunization programmes, allowable medical procedures and so on). The difference in the context of COVID-19 is, of course, that while all those data-gathering, measurement, assessment and risk determination activities *normally* fall into the background of the everyday machinery of governance and administration, government intervention in risk in the pandemic became an everyday public sphere event, a spectacle of politicians making statements, medical authorities and chief health officers fronting the media, epidemiologists becoming celebrities: all of these people explaining population risk, answering journalistic queries about risk and attempting to dispel the disinformation, distrust, protest and ignorance I described above. Managing risk at the level of population rather than the individual was suddenly the key talking point across much of the first years of the pandemic, and this was part of the 'strangeness' of living through the crisis.

The aporia of individualized and biopolitical risk frameworks was, then, partly responsible for providing the conditions in which concerns and suspicion about the range of COVID-19 vaccinations created greater hesitancy and disavowal than we might otherwise have expected among a population desperate to return to mobility and sociality, and this conceptualization provides an explanatory perspective for why some rather ludicrous disinformation, distrust and protest held appeal for some people. We can take this perspective on risk to a deeper level, too, to consider how the everydayness of risk management encourages not merely acceptance, hesitancy or disavowal of the vaccination programme, but encourages a relationship with vaccines (as with everything else) that is framed by the performative act of calculation.

Dyani Lewis (2022b: 51–2) points out that while many of the anti-vaccination lobby and protest groups were very clearly opposed to the mandating or, indeed, taking of any of the available vaccines, they distanced themselves strategically from the anti-vaxxer label. Instead, alongside their claims that mainstream media was distorting decision-making by refusing to carry anti-vaccination perspectives or the anecdotal and unsubstantiated stories of vaccine injuries and deaths, they claimed to 'encourage curiosity' in order to help people make their own decisions in weighing up the risk of catching COVID-19 and inoculations the risk of being vaccinated. As the anti-vaccine rhetoric of such groups became more sophisticated, they underscored the anecdotal stories with a quantification (often false) of vaccine risks. Such statistical quantification, then, competed with the existing quantification of COVID-19 risk that circulated so heavily in media and government releases since the start of the pandemic (Milan 2020). Of course, such quantification was unhelpful in performing a genuine calculation of the risk, particularly when members of the anti-vaccination lobby and protest groups have continued to refer to the mRNA vaccines as inoculations untested despite the quantified knowledge that they are now more tested in real-world settings than most other pharmaceutical solutions (Reuters Fact Check 2022).

To make a calculation of risk is to conduct a performative act that, retroactively, sustains the performance of the subject. However, as with all performativity of selfhood, calculation involves utilizing the practices, resources, rituals and frameworks that are made available in discourse. When making a responsible calculation (such as that it would be more responsible to *wait* until a greater number have been vaccinated because that would be a responsible way to treat the body), a calculation is made based on the normative ways in which we rehearse all risk decisions. When the shared needs of the public have, through decades of neoliberal and right-wing populist discourses, been positioned as an object of disdain and whereby responsibility is directed towards selfhood and personal gain (Butler and Athanasiou 2013: 105), it seems or *feels* not only responsible but ethically right. This is not to suggest that such an individualizing discourse of risk calculation is in any way hegemonic, since clearly very large numbers of people were vaccinated including many who did not wish to be for themselves but did so through knowledge that it may minimize risk for others more vulnerable (Attwell, Ward and Tomkinson 2021). Rather, it is to argue that the act of calculating risk operates in ways which are not fully in the control or agency of those making that calculation, and in some cases that is a calculation that is framed by a problematic individualism rather than a recognition of the interdependent sociality to which we are all ethically obliged.

Conclusion

The era of COVID-19 vaccination came after eighteen months of difficult, complex and sometimes painful health measures to manage and reduce the risk of spreading the virus, and was thereby welcomed by many, including those who might otherwise be apprehensive about the speed at which many of the vaccines were developed, tested, approved and made available, and among those who remain rightly suspicious of corporate pharmaceutical companies that profit from the development of health remedies. The advent of COVID vaccination was a difficult one for those billions who endured the mild-to-moderate side effects, or those whose hesitancy and refusal positioned them to be marginalized, lose employment or suffer family breakdowns through disagreement. However, vaccination heralded such a significant change to the conditions of risk and liveability and the cultural practices through which we had been managing risk in many parts of the world that, as with other aspects of the pandemic, warrants a process of mourning that which is lost – the lockdowns, the social distancing – no matter how difficult such a situation was felt to be.

A failure to mourn adequately, as we know from Freud (1994), leaves us unable to work through and incorporate change and loss into our futural selfhood as a form of transformation, and at risk of falling into melancholia which acts as an attack of the self on the self, and at risk of losses of self-esteem and the willingness to live. I will discuss the operations of mourning and melancholia in greater detail in Chapter 8, but it is worth noting here that an inability to mourn the advent of COVID vaccination creates difficulties among not only those who turn to vaccine refusal but among those of us who were happily vaccinated but needed thereby to experience a substantial change to the – by then – familiar norms of protecting ourselves and others from the virus through other means. In other words, it was not as simple as a return to normativity, not only because the pandemic persists in such a way that the prior norm is a nostalgic memory, but also because no sudden change to cultural practices of sociality occurs without the need to recognize that change as the loss of a past and a transformation of identity, relationality and belonging to proceed into the future.

I have addressed in this chapter some of the ways in which vaccine hesitancy and refusal was conditioned by new forms of disinformation, populist distrust, communitarianism among protest groups and the culturally produced condition of ignorance, and that underlying the appeal of such discourses and practices is the way in which we have been conditioned in Western neoliberal cultures to perceive risk as an individualized activity of calculation rather than a matter for governance. I also wrote earlier that there was no value in further polarizing the pro- and anti- (or hesitant) vaccine groups, slamming ignorance or criticizing those who have been misled by disinformation and a culture of distrust is not only going to fail to increase vaccination rates, but is unethical when such persons are not fully responsible for the conditions that positioned them to embrace a hesitancy or refusal discourse. Developing ways in which risk can be better understood not as a calculation for the individual but as something which is shared across an interdependent community is not only a way to return to the importance of mutual welfare, but a protective force against vaccine refusal when we are next dependent as a whole on its uptake.

8

Disrupted futurity: Mourning the self and the other

Introduction

A common complaint emerging during the second year of the pandemic among, particularly, younger people was that the COVID-19 pandemic and the related health restrictions took away a sense of future. This was often expressed in relation to increased anxiety during periods in which schools and universities required students to study from home (Lucas et al. 2021) and regularly framed future in terms of social life, relationships and employment. Often, the experience of young people through lockdowns, mask-wearing, disrupted social lives and education, delays moving out of their parents' homes and postponing travel and other normative 'rituals' of the transition to adulthood (Hickey-Moody 2016) was encapsulated with phrases such as 'many young people now face an uncertain future' (Topsfield 2021), often ignoring the fact that certain futures were not necessarily common among young people before the pandemic. To point to the experience of younger people is to note that the kinds of 'disruptions' to everyday cultural practices owing to the pandemic and the regulatory measures taken to protect lives are experienced by different people in different ways, including affecting how a construction of 'futurity' – which I argue here is a core element in identity performativity – is perceived.

A common response in some media, parts of the blogosphere and made by high-profile, older celebrity opinion-makers has been to argue that this was an expected response from young people because they 'lack resilience' (O'Connor 2020, Qasi 2020, Topsfield and Aubrey 2022). This ill-considered response tends not only to ignore the substantial evidence about young people's actual, measured resilience (Harvey 2012), or their own perception of personal resilience and resilience among their peers in discussing their strategies of coping with the constraints of lockdown, immobility and other social distancing measures

(Hall and Dexter 2021), it also ignores the substantial diversity among young people's personal assets for coping with changed circumstances, disruptions and the expectations of future well-being, and how these are often demarcated along lines of gender, geography and socio-economic determinants.

Framing the experiences of young people in terms of a disrupted sense of futurity and diverse experiences of resilience opens valuable questions as to how normative, health and stable subjectivities among the wider public operate in terms of temporal trajectories not merely into coherence with the past (Butler 1990), but also into the future along lines of what is sometimes referred to as 'chrononormativities' or 'institutionally and culturally enforced rhythms, or timings, [that] shape flesh into legible, acceptable embodiment' (Freeman 2010: 4). As subjects who perform our identities in the context of temporalities, we are constituted in ways which call upon us to imagine a future direction of selfhood, social participation and belonging. As I argue below, a blow to the chrononormative practices of futural thinking – the uncertainty of what will happen, who we will be, how we will participate and where we belong – demands not merely resilience to critically engage with the complex relationship between identity and temporality. It also calls upon us to mourn the disrupted or 'lost' futural trajectory in ways that are necessary, lest that mourning not be achieved and instead result in a debilitating melancholia. What we learn from the statements about futurity made by younger people is instructive for all whose lives were disrupted by the pandemic.

I begin this chapter with a brief discussion of futurity, chrononormativity and identity to demonstrate how a normative temporal approach or trajectory is significant for the production and performance of a stable sense of identity – albeit never quite universally or democratically shared. I would then like to further the discussion on young people and resilience in the context of disrupted temporality, returning to some of the points made in the introduction to this book about the different approaches to resilience that inform how we respond to the disruption of the pandemic. I will then discuss how we can understand practices of coping with the lost sense of future through psychoanalytic approaches to mourning and melancholia, whereby the change or rupture not only in expectation but in ordinary, chrononormative patterns of identity performance must be mourned – and that recognizing the need to mourn what is lost is the key to a critical resilience that can guide us through future population health crises.

Chrononormativity, futurity and identity

The fact that identity is performative, constituted in language and practised by the coherent and intelligible reiteration of norms, signifiers, behaviours, tastes and attitudes means it is always a regulated process without an end or a final becoming (Butler 1990: 70, 145). This approach to understanding identity, subjectivity and selfhood implies a context of time – a subject is constituted in the encounter and engagement with discourses, cultural practices, languages and regulatory norms, and in that engagement is persistently in a process of becoming and flux. However, the subject is simultaneously called upon and obliged by the cultural demands for coherence, intelligibility and recognizability *over time*, such that past shifts in identity must be explained and future changes, adjustments and slippages minimized or – at least – provided a grounding for an explanation that fits in with those demands for coherence and self-unity.

At the same time, a substantial aspect of identity performativity is a sense of futurity. Futurity is significantly connected with liveability – it is not necessarily a liveable life without a sense that that life has a future. A vast range of cultural frameworks and practices actively encourage a sense of futurity as a part of the performativity of the now: a temporal trajectory that pre-empts and plans for the future, connected with concepts of hope, aspiration, survival and pleasure. For example, in many parts of the world young adults are called upon to plan for a happy retirement by participating in superannuation and pension schemes; a normative life of good citizenship often involves planning for the payment of debt; we mostly undertake study and training with a sense of future employment prospects (and sometimes just to gain knowledge that will be useful in the future rather than merely pleasurable to engage with today). We put away funds to pay for future holidays, homes or to plan for survival, despite the ways in which a financial debt culture has encouraged us to disavow future finances in order to make an immediate purchase or (Lazzarato 2011). And, of course, during the early years of the COVID-19 pandemic, some people participated in 'panic buying' of foods and toilet paper – indicating not merely a concern about future availability, but to maximizing future survival and hygiene. Many of us have had COVID-19 vaccinations and boosters with an eye to reducing the chances of infection in the future.

In other words, the performance and practice of identity is governed in part by a futural orientation made intelligible through a variety of framings of temporality. Elizabeth Freeman (2010: 3) introduced the concept of chrononormativity to describe the ways in which practices, behaviours and identities are organized through the use of time. Freeman understands chrononormativity as a form of institutional and cultural implantation whereby forces and regulatory measures come to feel like binding somatic and embodied facts. These include such everyday artefacts and experiences as calendars, schedules, seasons, school bells, embodied normative processes at dawn and dusk, ways of being in the night as opposed to how one performs identity in the daylight, and the use of years to mark the passage of time and the relationship between the length of time one has been alive (their age) and the practices of subjectivity and selfhood that are not only expected but willingly adopted and sometimes even regimented (a 'retirement age'; an age of availability for military service, and so on). Or it is the framing factor in what Foucault (2008: 226) identified as the disposition of the contemporary subject of neoliberal societies to become 'entrepreneurs of the self' – that is, where neoliberalism becomes the logic that infuses all aspects of society and subjectivity, one invests in the self through processes of continued betterment oriented towards a futural outcome or the protection against risks in the future. For John Urry (2007: 98), following Lefebvre, *lived time* comes to dominate subjectivity: 'Time becomes a resource, differentiated off from social space, consumed, deployed and exhausted' under the domination of clock time (98), serving as the means by which we regulate ourselves through patterns of bodily use that produce identities in relation to work, careers, entertainment choices, leisure, health and play (Munt 2002).

Chrononormativity does more, however, than simply regulate the individual body into a particular pattern that fosters sometimes problematic requirements of productivity. It is simultaneously oriented towards the interdependency among subjects that binds communities and populations to norms. This, of course, emerges historically. As historian E.P. Thompson (1967) noted, although the introduction of the church clock in fourteenth-century Europe made time measurement widely available, with subsequent shifts whereby private clocks and watches were turned from luxuries to everyday conveniences, the purpose of clock-time by the Industrial Revolution was to synchronize a public in order to enhance labour's productivity and efficiency over every-wider spaces, producing what we now perceive as a form of global time (Castells 2000: 463). This synchronization became, of course, a form of chrononormativity by the twenty-first century in which normative practices of temporality, planning, perceptions of the past and considerations of futurity infuse identity practices as an element of intelligible social participation and belonging.

Here is where we can consider for school-aged young people (as well as many working adults) the ways in which pandemic-related health regulations upset the normativity of time in ways which impinge on the alignment of performative identity and chrononormative temporality. The knowable routine of the school day and the weekend, of the daily chore of travel to school by the appointed hour, the periodization of the day, the after-school activities, the evening homework, and so on, are all disciplinary measures that work with temporal norms to produce docile subjects (Foucault 1977). As subjects, we naturally have a passionate attachment to that normality and docility as the very things that constitute our subjectivity in subordination (Butler 1997: 7, 27). To lose those everyday temporal disciplines in a shift to home-schooling, online classes, the removal of the need for travel to school and, most particularly, the consistency, shaping and framing of selfhood, belonging and sociality these temporal disciplines bring is to disrupt the self, once again calling upon subjectivity to be re-framed and shaped in unfamiliar ways.

This is to think about the disruption of the everyday temporality that governs and disciplines us through the familiarity of everyday clock time, but what about the perception of the everyday to come – the shift in expectation and futurity? Here it is not the loss of familiar and regular temporal routines but the gain of a less-easily knowable future. Futurity is often tied up with aspiration, which itself cannot be disconnected from the temporality of subjectivity as, in part, a future-oriented process. For Arjun Appadurai (2003) aspiration is not simply individual wants that govern choices, but is actively formed in interaction within social life – what is significant, the materiality of certain social expectations, the uneven capacity to aspire and the inequitable distribution of material and psychological resources that give some people confidence their aspirations will be met while others have the certainty that aspirations are fruitless. We might consider here, then, the processes of chrononormativity to be a considerable part of the social formation of aspiration that is futurally oriented – the knowability of certain expectations and life milestones. Again, for a student (some, not all, of course), we could point to futural and aspirational markers such as graduation from school, acceptance into tertiary study, a few months of leisure, the first entry into bars, clubs and drinking at parties, serious relationships, the expectation of future employment. As chrononorms that shape an aspirational 'expectation' of opportunities and choices in a futural trajectory of a life, these govern aspects of the performativity of subjecthood, driving particular behaviours, the labour of study, the persistence through difficult times and the attitude or orientation towards hope.

For Joseph Pugliese (2004), such orientation towards expectations of the future has significance for liveability and well-being. The form of temporality experienced by those who cannot have a sense as to how long they may endure an adverse condition of life is, then, a violence done unto subjectivity. Using the example of the asylum seeker detained on arrival in a new country (for unknowable and in many cases severely protracted periods), Pugliese puts the unknowability of futurity this way:

> The present weighs down life in its own immovable immanence, where the only hope for movement resides in flashbacks, backward to the very traumas that the refugee had so desperately desired to escape. Symmetrically, to flash-forward into the future is to generate more trauma, specifically the fear and anxiety of deportation back to the persecution from which the refugee had originally fled. The refugee's life is violently circumscribed by these two polar bookends: the trauma of the past / the trauma of the future.
>
> (299)

Futurity, as the very thing that 'gives meaning and hope', was actively eradicated from the labour experience of a young, middle-class person experiencing lockdown, immobility or social distancing protocols that disrupt the normative sense of what they may expect to experience in the performativity of growing into adulthood. It is, of course, immaterial if those experiences are primarily going to parties, bars or clubs, attending one's graduation, entering the workforce, beginning tertiary education or spending a gap year overseas. Or merely 'having available' a range of Western, middle-class opportunities to choose. It is the fact of these being *held off* with no clear, knowable date on which regular, normative lifecycle milestones can be passed that fragments a sense of futurity and therefore a sense of linear subjectivity.

The lack of futurity in an indeterminate experience of interrupted lifecycle can be described as a form of *forced temporality* external to the normative temporalities of performative identities conditioned by the expectations, planning, theatrics of unknowable futures, financial security, pleasure, relationships and social belonging. If a liveable life is constituted in social participation and belonging that is conditional on the intelligible and (relatively) normative performance of coherent subjectivity, then those experiencing a lost sense of future pleasures, securities or liveability are unable to participate in what is *recognized* as normativity by virtue of being unable to articulate a selfhood through temporal concepts of lifecycle and ageing. For those without access to the resources through which to perform an alternative intelligibility of identity, exacerbated by the desire to belong to a new, safe or secure environment at home away from the risk of the virus, the conditions for liveability remain unmet. This, obviously for many younger people, is made more problematic by the fact that health resilience among the young is relatively higher than their older peers, meaning the disruption of futurity is in favour of the protection of others (ethically sound in a world of interdependency, but ethics does not mean the maximization of pleasures of freedoms for individuals). While the liminal experience of disrupted normative temporality can, for some subjects, clearly produce a communal equality that enhances resilience and supportive belonging, a lack of knowable futurity can, for others, exacerbate marginalization.

Young people, resilience and future liveability

Resilience involves a sense of futurity or 'hope' for a pleasing, enjoyable, safe and survivable future. At the same time, however, resilience is a necessary component of coping with the disruption to a future. As I noted in the introduction, resilience has been a key trope in discussions as to how individuals and whole populations have 'managed' survival and liveability across the pandemic. There, I pointed out that there are two different approaches to resilience: a psychological approach that tends to perceive resilience as an individual trait (sometimes innate) and practised alone, and what is known as the 'social ecology' of resilience approach, which recognizes that resilience is fostered in the intersection between personal capabilities and the ecology in which that person is placed, including familial, institutional and peer-networked resources and infrastructures (Unger 2012b). In other words, while the former 'locates' resilience within the individual, the latter see resilience in the context of interdependency which, as I have argued throughout this book, is a key component of recognizing the significance of subjectivity in the context of a pandemic that, itself, takes advantage of human interdependency as an *a priori* fact of liveability and survival.

Both approaches to resilience, however, have a tendency to build on concepts in which *norms* are seen as the measure of a resilient subject or setting. Normative life 'milestones', for example, are used as measures of the extent to which a resilient subject overcomes adversity: educational graduation, self-esteem scores, absence of substance use/abuse (Wexler et al. 2009: 566). Indeed, the articulation of 'positive development under stress' (Unger 2012b: 15) constitutes an instance of resilience's conceptual location within normativities, whether the concept is used in the psychological or social ecological models. Measures are, of course, a necessity if one is attempting to account for resilience. However, the deployment of norms as universal measures is problematic as they figure certain actions or behaviours that a subject may utilize as coping practices as non-normative and non-resilient. For example, sleep, laziness and unwillingness to leave the house are often considered traits of depression (Kendall-Tackett 2017), and the use of illicit recreational drugs is often presented as a sign of non-resilience; acts of graffiti are represented as an indicator of a poorly adjusted individual. However, for some subjects, these acts in themselves can be formations of resilience and creative strategies for coping with adversities. In other words, in thinking about resilience, we need to be very careful not to presume norms and measure people by them, but to recognize that antinormative behaviours may sometimes be performances of resistance that foster resilience (Wiegman and Wilson 2015).

In this respect, on the one hand, certain practices in relation to everyday chrononormativities might be mis-perceived as evidence of a non-resilient young person – sleeping during the day, remaining awake overnight, spending large amounts of time playing digital games, and so on. On the other hand, if we take a more 'critical' approach to resilience that disavows norms as the measure of a resilient subject, we can see that those same practices can very well be formations of resilience for others, precisely because they are anti-normative. Sleeping more or, conversely, not getting enough sleep (Illingworth et al. 2022) may well have been protective factors or formations of resilience. In this respect, it is important not to assume that the behaviours reported about young people were necessarily always indications of a lack of resilience or, indeed, a lack of well-being and healthy disposition, but may well have been practices adopted for survival and liveability in the context of a disrupted or delayed sense of futurity and the re-framing that causes for subjectivity itself.

I pointed out in Chapter 4 that there were many false claims that the lockdowns in many countries were causing very high rates of suicide. These claims, on the whole, turned out to be false, scurrilous disinformation used for political purposes and in anti-lockdown protest speech. In that chapter, I argued that one explanation for this is the fact that the shared experience of adversity served, as is often the case, as a protective factor. It is *probable* that a number of youth suicides that may have occurred were prevented not only by the protective factor of the shared experience of adversity but also the lack of opportunity that may arise when a young person is stuck in the supervision-setting of a family household every day and night. However, it is known that in many jurisdictions, there was an increase by young people (especially teenagers) in the use of suicide prevention supports, such as telephone and online counselling services (OECD 2021).

Understanding why this increase in the use of counselling and support is complex and requires substantial quantitative and qualitative research across a wide range of jurisdictions. However, rather than presuming a lack of resilience is cause, or that the growth of discourse on mental health predisposes young people to seek support in ways that did not occur in earlier years, we can hypothesize that a loss of sense of aspiration and hopefulness that is part of the identity practice oriented towards futurity may have been in many cases a lost sense of liveability. Lost futurity means a lost capacity to perceive or achieve aspirations, particularly in the 'strange temporality' of the daily cycles of non-futurity in the pandemic months before vaccines brought hope for a change in regulated immobility.

Hopelessness is a key factor in much of the contemporary academic discussion of mental health risk in general and is sometimes used as a predictor for recognizing suicidal behaviour (Battin 1995: 13), although it is also particularly associated with suicidality among teenagers. Hopelessness is usually understood as despair or desperateness, the lack of expectation of a future situation or goal one desires or feels one should desire. For Holden and colleagues (1989: 500), hopelessness is counter to social desirability, which is understood as the capacity to describe oneself in terms by which society judges a person as legitimate or desirable. Psychological and psychiatric measurement techniques frequently rely on Aaron T. Beck's (1974) Hopelessness Scale, which utilizes a twenty-question true/false survey designed to measure feelings about the future, expectation and self-motivation in adults over the age of seventeen years as a predictor of suicidal behaviour. However, from a cultural theory perspective, hopelessness can be understood as *affective* in relation to aspirations for belonging – whether that is a felt sense of attachment to others or, more pertinently, to the normativity through which a futurity is performative and a selfhood can be articulated in terms of temporal lifecycles, expected milestones and so on. Hopelessness is not the *lack* or *loss* of perceiving a future, but a particular attachment to a perceived future that is undesirable, which may include in this circumstance a perceived future of protracted lockdown and social distancing, a perceived disruption to the available employment or study options, a perceived curtailment of the long-awaited post-schooling social existence some expect as a young adult.

Nevertheless, it is important not to assume that hopelessness was a universal youth experience during the early years of the pandemic. Rather, there is emerging evidence from the UK that a substantial number of young people reported feeling happier, better adjusted and more comfortable with themselves and their identities during the lockdown periods (Soneson et al. 2022), and again we could consider this in terms of the power of the shared experience of adversity in producing resilience rather than annihilating it. In other words, there is substantial diversity in the distribution and capability of resilience to face the adversity of a disrupted sense of aspiration, hope and futurity, and the forms of resilience themselves are more diverse. Here, then, it is necessary to avoid claims about youth resilience but to recognize that the skills, capabilities, peer-networks, ecological supports, critical capacities and other resources that constitute, foster and sustain resilience are unevenly available. One of those critical capabilities I would like to turn to in the next section is the ability to recognize the need to mourn a lost sense of futurity – altered expectations – in order to survive that adjustment or rupture *as* a loss.

Into the pandemic: Mourning the lost future

When a chrononormative practice such as a lived everyday temporality or an orientation towards the expectations of a future are radically disrupted, altered without agency or perceived as lost, they must be mourned. Indeed, mourning is central to the stable practices of the psyche and, hence, to subjectivity in both individual and interrelational terms. We might consider here, for example, that the immobility mandated as a health measure in the first two years of the pandemic prevented not only the routine for young people of being among peers and friends who support resilience, but (i) the disruption to the disciplinary framework of everyday chrononormative times to which one has an attachment as that which produces certain aspects of subjectivity, and (ii) the loss of an anticipated or knowable futurity as that which constitutes elements of performativity. While these are disruptions, ruptures, alterations or reduced capacities for aspiration, these shifts are losses – and that requires mourning which, as I argue, is key to resilience.

Mourning is not, however, an inherent practice we simply 'do' or know how to do. It is a learned capability that depends on the kind of resilience I described above in order to be performed. Writing during the First World War, Sigmund Freud (1994) introduced a psychoanalytic framework to understand the two different processes of dealing with loss. Mourning, for Freud, is a conscious response to dealing with the grief involved in the loss of a loved object (which may be a person, a situation, a practice or a material thing to which one has an attachment). Melancholia involves an unconscious practice of grieving for a loss that cannot be fully comprehended or recognized. Both involve departures from 'the normal attitude to life' (243) and both are painful experiences of feelings of dejection, 'cessation of interest in the outside world' and a turning away of the possibilities of replacing that loss with an alternative attachment (244). However, they are distinguished by the fact that mourning involves a conscious recognition that can be worked through the meanings and implications of that loss and coming to terms with the changed environment in which the object of attachment is absent. Melancholia, however, is pathological whereby the subject cannot process the loss, turning instead towards a diminishing of self-regard and a substantial impoverishment of the ego – feelings of worthlessness that cannot be explained and worked through in the unconscious.

The distinction is significant for making sense of how people respond differently to the loss of chrononormative frameworks of everyday temporality and aspirational futurity. The sudden change to temporal routines that give a subject of sense of identity, discipline or meaning must be mourned, just as the lost futurity, aspiration or certainty in the future must be mourned. As with all mourning, this involves what Butler (2004: 21), building on Freud from a poststructuralist perspective, identified as accepting the loss by undergoing or 'submitting' to a 'transformation' of the self. That is, because the 'I' or 'self' is never fully separate from those others or objects to which one has an attachment and ties that constitute us, there is no possibility of restoration or seeing mourning as a temporary measure – the prior order will never quite return and the self must change in order for the mourning to be complete. If the chrononormative order and the aspiration of futurity are constitutive of our subjectivities, and they are, then their loss in the regulatory practices of pandemic suppression require mourning in order to undergo that transformation of the self.

For those who can rationalize the rupture to chrononormative frameworks of being, belonging and sociality by recognizing that a permanent transformation of the self is necessary, then mourning is possible. However, this is where critical capabilities as one aspect of resilience come into play – the ability to bounce back, somewhat different, from the shock of the change to those chrononormative regimes and the alteration of a sense of futurity. Part of the argument I am making here is that the resources to enable that conscious mourning are not evenly or democratically available to all subjects (and given these are resources acquired both culturally and psychically over time, I am suggesting that some young people may have a greater likelihood of needing further time to develop these fully). What we have, then, is the possibility of melancholia – the inability to work through that uncertainty and change in order to recognize what has been lost. As with other social changes that need to be mourned, those that cannot will deny it, repress it or otherwise generate unconscious responses that lead to a melancholic attack on the self (La Caze 2011). It brings about a decrease in self-esteem (Butler 1997: 184) that thereby overthrows the drive for to cling to life itself (Butler 2006: 119).

Thinking about melancholia helps to explain the psychic pain many young people experienced according to the substantial increase in counselling calls and, of course, through no fault of their own or no 'lack' in personal resilience but a lack of the critical capabilities necessary to recognize the loss of chrononormative attachments as a loss that must be mourned. Melancholia also helps explain some of the practices of COVID-deniers who, fuelled by disinformation, were able to find a self-destructive world-view of conspiracy upon which they could adhere, disavowing the need for mourning. The key indication here, then, is that better resources to mourn change and the sudden advent of unknowability are needed beyond ordinary advocation of stoicism and persistence in adversity. Calls for better resilience should be read, then, as calls for better resources for critically recognizing the impact of chrononormative losses on identity itself and, therefore, creating the conditions in which those losses can be mourned as a necessary transformation of selfhood.

It might also be remarked here that one additional condition in which mourning is required is to assist in the adjustment to the end of pandemic suppression measures, the advent of vaccination as a solution (always only partial) to the pandemic and the return to certain forms of mobility and social behaviours.

While these may *appear* to be a 'return to normality' – a phrase widely used as regulatory measures eased at various times and in various regions (e.g. Brown 2022, Council of the European Union 2022) – they are themselves ruptures of new norms that, once again, change the chrononormative framework that constitutes and sustains us. In other words, a return to being able to plan for the future, a return to the clock time framework of leaving for work or school in the morning involves another rupture, once that also requires us to mourn the attachments that have been lost, no matter how painful those attachments such as lockdowns and social distancing may have been for some. We become attached to the altered norms not because they give us pleasure or happiness or safety or survival, but because they constitute our transformed subjectivity through their new regimes of temporality. When they too are gone, there may be substantial relief and jubilation (such as the partying on 'Freedom Day' in the UK – one way in which to process change) but they also must be recognized as loss and mourned, even if that form of mourning is not one marked by sadness, sorrow and self-pity.

Conclusion

Contemporary formations of individualism tend to disavow the significance of the ecological setting in which we are thrown and which, through interrelationality and interdependence, constitute our subjectivity. Chrononormativities such as everyday clock time regimentation and thinking that is futurally oriented towards expectation and planning are a key part of that ecology and deploy various cultural and psychic formations such as discipline and aspiration to produce us and govern the performativity of our identities in ways that help meet the cultural demand for intelligibility. The COVID-19 pandemic disrupted our practices of time very substantially, and this was probably more marked for young, school-aged people whose time is typically more regimented and regularized than others, and who are encouraged to think in futural terms about a time beyond the institutional setting of school life. Where claims about young people's lacking resilience were used to counter some of the public knowledge of an increase in the use of online and telephone counselling support – or where those figures were used to suggest that the health measures were inappropriately harsh – a significant point has been missed about how we might better perceive the kinds of resilience that allow identities to persist and stabilize through the adversity of sudden, unwanted and unknowable change.

By recognizing that changes to temporal frameworks of the kind experienced in this pandemic are also to be perceived as an irrecoverable (rather than merely 'temporary') loss, we are better placed to recognize the value of practices of mourning. This is not necessarily to suggest that health authorities around the globe should have accompanied COVID-19 safety and self-protection advice with leaflets and webpages that describe a critical theory of chrononormativity and a psychoanalytic discourse of mourning and melancholia (although these may, for some, have been useful). Rather, it is to suggest that if we want to protect a population from the negative mental health consequences of very necessary and well-recognized population health measures of quarantine, lockdown, social distancing and other practices that actively protect lives, hospital infrastructures and the well-being of front-line health workers, then we need to consider how resilience can be better fostered by greater critical skills that help people – including the very young – to rationalize change as loss, and to thereby undergo mourning rather than fall into the melancholia that comes from an inability to recognize loss.

Conclusion: COVID futures – Ethical care in interdependency

Introduction

In the Introduction to this book, and repeatedly throughout, I have drawn attention to two key frameworks that help us make sense of identity in the COVID years: the shift in everydayness that can be figured as a major cultural rupture, and the incompatibility of two different practices of social resilience: an individualist one and one which is grounded in recognizing and drawing on the inherent interdependency that constitutes all social beings. The disruption of the first and the renewed attention to the second in media, communication and public sphere discourse has shifted the constitutive frameworks that make everyday self-identity intelligible and coherent to ourselves and others. Managing that process of a change in the grounding of identity has, for some, required acts of mourning the lost past, the shifted expectations and aspirations of the future, and the changed practices of everyday mobility, touch, comportment and other aspects of performing identity in the face of sociality.

In this short conclusion, I would like to make a few remarks about how the disruption of the pandemic has opened opportunities to better utilize that inherent interdependency in practices of care, and how some of those opportunities have been disregarded as we move into what some jurisdictions refer to as an 'end to COVID exceptionalism' or as 'COVID normal' – that is, recognizing that the virus is now an incurable condition of living and surviving on the planet. While there has been, therefore, a substantial cultural transformation, the opportunities to produce a more ethical practice of social engagement grounded in the mutuality of care risk being lost if the future of the pandemic is perceived only as a return to 'normal', as that 'normal' implies all the social inequities and disadvantages that distributed vulnerability to disease differentially across class, age and global region. To put this as a question: if our identities are re-shaped and re-constituted by the disruptive experience of the pandemic, then in what ways might the foregrounding of an alternative, more ethical interdependency be drawn upon to produce more ethical selves, actions, behaviours and ways-of-being that are oriented towards recognizing our ethical obligations to those with whom we cohabit the planet in all its futural precarity? I will start with a return to interdependency by discussing it in the context of care and equitable access to care, followed by some thoughts on what it means to move into a post-pandemic phase of normativity and whether or not the learnings from COVID-19 include a greater appreciation of our interdependency not just with one another, but with a wider ecology.

Care in equitable interdependency

Being a contemporary subject means being constituted in an unavoidable interdependency with others, despite the social, cultural and institutional forces that attempt to shape identity into a radical individuality that often calls upon people to consider their needs, desires and means of being satisfied in ways that are competitive with – and sometimes adversarial towards – others. Across this book, I have drawn on and discussed many instances in which interdependency has come into conflict with radical claims and attempted practices of independence, selfishness, assertions of sovereignty and agency over one's own health at the cost of others, the differentials between social and individual management of risk, and so on. Critical and scholarly engagement with ethics of sociality, however, has persistently pointed to the ethical benefits of eschewing individualist thinking that has dominated liberal-humanist and neoliberal frameworks of contemporary being, and this has been particularly apparent in post-structuralist and feminist theorizing, both of which offer alternative knowledge frameworks for relationality based in the mutuality of care.

Such a framework often draws on Foucault's analysis of older models of care and subjectivity. In his histories of the practices of subjectivity, Foucault (2005) identified the care of the self as an early philosophical formulation found in early Greek, Hellenistic and Roman philosophy and Christian spirituality. In the practice of caring for the self, it is care for the other – other people – that is indispensable in achieving the goal of mastery of the self (127). In caring well for the self, one seeks to care for others whereby the practice of the self and subjectivity is seen always as part of an ethical social relationship (164). Although dislodged in European culture by the approaches to reason credited to Descartes (14) and more broadly within European Enlightenment culture which continues to dominate perceptions of ethics and selfhood into twenty-first-century liberal and neoliberal modernity, the ancient model of the care of the self as articulated by Foucault provides a powerful framework for ethical relations today. Instances of such ethics can, of course, be found in many localized cultural settings, even if this is not a dominant framework in the neoliberal, Euro-centric formations of sociality. Such an ethics is thus not built on emphasizing the 'do nots' (do not get infected, do not infect others) but on articulating articulate decision-making and negotiation as core aspects of subjectivity, belonging and relationality.

COVID-19 as a health issue or health crisis draws attention to care, but that is not to say that in itself it should be the principal object of care. By making an issue of care, we would be hiving it off from the wider and more important issues of ethical subjectivity built in mutual care and relationality. Rather, an ethics of care grounded in relationality and directed towards the other is one which overcomes the traditional attempts to bound issues of care from other social issues, from phallogocentric frameworks that divide private care from public care, and from the institutionalization of care which relegates it to the health and medical professions and ignores the substantial performative role it must play in an ethics across the everyday (Brugère 2019). Indeed, considering care and ethics together warrants bringing the more marginalized practices of everyday care to the centre not of health and medical issues, but to relationality itself – acts of 'caring with' that can more democratically meet the needs of ensuring that each subject in interrelationality with each other is cared about and safe from the infection of a dangerous virus (Tronto 2013). This is the key learning from the differential treatment of subjects in our interdependent and cohabited social world, and yet the biopolitical and population health models that provide one of the dominant lenses by which we make sense of the experience of COVID-19 in media and communication regularly eschews opportunities to consider how risk is experienced diversely. For example, we know (but don't often discuss) there are some who are more at risk of mortality from COVID-19 – even in the post-vaccination era – such as people of lower socio-economic status, the global poor, people who are precariously employed or without stable housing, people who live in conditions of war or climate catastrophe, the lower echelons of underpaid health workers and the elderly in inadequate care settings (The Care Collective

2020: 1). They are *not* more at risk because of the way the virus attacks the body, although that is of course part of the picture. They are more at risk due to the existing undemocratically distributed frameworks and infrastructures of care that leave some people more precarious and less grievable than others (Butler 2009: 28). And these are the neoliberal practices, structures and discourses that abandon some subjects as 'bare life' while others are 'cared about'.

This spirals out not merely from the medical concerns about what SARS-CoV-2 does to some bodies that exempt other (fitter, younger and better cared-for) bodies. Rather, the differential distribution of care was witnessed across an array of inequitable experiences of the protective health measure. Where I spent my time in Melbourne, Australia, during the first two years of the pandemic – often in the context of one of the world's longest periods of lockdown and mobility restriction – I witnessed the sad reality of the inequitable distribution of the impact of the vital and necessary health measures, and how that experience emphatically aligned with existing inequities. From the privileged position of being able to gaze out of the top-floor window on the south of my townhouse, I was able to see some of the elite inner-urban buildings, with couples drinking champagne on their balconies during periods of lockdown. From the north side, however, I looked onto the crammed apartments of social housing towers where the virus was known to have spread quickly among inhabitants, many of whom were crammed into small rooms. Surveillance helicopters, and the lights and sirens of regular police patrols marked a stark contrast between how the 'disruption' of the pandemic was experienced – an image of affluent comfort and an image of hell. And that, of course, is just one anecdotal, local example in the context of what was visually available, and does not account for the massive discrepancies across different jurisdictions, classes and regions of the world where, in some cases, infrastructure to prevent viral spread simply does not exist, the ability to map rates of infections lags behind the resources of other countries and the capability to distribute vaccines once available has remained poor. It is not at all unreasonable to argue that of the six-and-a-half million COVID deaths by late 2022, many of those deaths would have been prevented had there been a more equitable distribution of care – more 'caring about' the marginalized other.

There are many other examples of the inequitable experience of the pandemic. Thankfully, in some cases, such inequities were treated as scandalous, such as the party at 10 Downing Street attended by senior staff in Prime Minister Boris Johnson's office in breach of the very rules they were enforcing upon the wider population in the UK (Reicher 2022), the insistence of tennis player Novak Djokovic on attempting to use legal measures to avoid the rule that required all visitors to Australia to be vaccinated (Sakkal and Koob 2022) and the squalid conditions of the precariously homed and people on disability pensions during the COVID lockdowns (e.g. Topsfield and Millar 2021). By becoming framed as scandals and generating outrage and shame, there is at least an indication that inequities are seen by many to be unacceptable, particularly during a period of crisis in which it was regularly stated that all human beings were facing this together. The reality, of course, is that some were facing the pandemic and its health protections with far greater comfort and resources than others.

If part of the learning, then, of the COVID years has been that we live and survive in an *a priori* interdependency, and that interdependency not only allows a virus to travel easily between subjects but also enables the survival of subjects, and also distributes that survival in inequitable ways, then the learning itself is fruitless if that interdependency is not experienced with greater equity. I have been discussing interdependency throughout much of this book as something that needs to be critically recognized not only if we are to understand the socio-cultural impact of the pandemic's disruption, but if we are to have more ethical lives oriented towards the other rather than individuated self. No subject, as we know, lives or survives outside of the interdependency and cohabitation with all other subjects, and the fact this interdependency is a condition of liveability that pre-exists our own, individualized subjectivity, we are ethically bound to act *without violence* to all others (Butler 2020). I have pointed out how that includes disavowing the violence of shaming those who refuse vaccination as much as the violence of ignoring health protection measures in a way that may infect others we do not know and will never meet. Managing the complex terrain of apprehending interdependency in our everyday lives does not, of course, warrant establishing more rules or measures about who is more ethical than another, since such mechanisms of calculation are always bound to create or sustain subordination and marginalization (although we do not, of course, want to do away with rules altogether). What it means, rather, is that attempting to live in ethical interdependency requires that we – as a global society – *listen* to the stories of others, whether that is the story of the person who insists they do not need to wear a mask, the story of the communities who deny the existence of SARS-CoV-2 or the stories of those young people who forge alternative and non-normative practices of resilience to cope with being locked in for months with their parents without respite. Listening is the starting point of developing relational interests and building the connections and engagement that foster a shared responsibility towards the collective (Dreher 2009). Indeed, even at the most practical level, there is a growing awareness that if some of the vaccine hesitant had been listened to rather than having their strange views on vaccination dismissed they would not have become militant refusers, protesters and spreaders of misinformation (Lewis 2022b: 108).

However important it is to act and perform our selfhood and subjectivity in ways which incorporate that interdependency, and to utilize this in more ethical practices of caring about one another, this is not to suggest that interdependency itself is the ethical goal. Rather, as Butler (2020: 40) has been pointed out, an ethics of non-violence based on interdependency demands an 'equal grievability of lives'. This is different from saying that all individuals are equal to one another, or have equal rights, but requires critiquing such individualism in favour of 'a more fully imagined interdependency … in new forms of civic and political life' (44). We might frame that in such a way as to understand equality in civic and political life means equitable access to care, broadly defined as caring about, for and with others (Tronto 2013) – obligatory forms of care that are practices of caring for the self and constituting the self.

Towards COVID-normal ecologies

The phrase 'COVID normal' began being used in Australia in late 2020 to describe the ideal situation of removed health restrictions such as immobility, mask-wearing and border restrictions, and living with the virus as a normal part of everyday life (Behind the News 2020). Across many jurisdictions around the world in the post-vaccination phase of the pandemic, the removal of restrictions has meant understanding that risk and precarity of the wider population will rise and fall in seasonal waves, that there may be grounds for new restrictions at times, but that on the whole an 'opening up' has occurred that restores the majority of everyday practices *as if* the pandemic and its difficult protection measures had not occurred (Lewis 2022b: 114). This is not to suggest that there is widespread disregard for the pandemic and the social and cultural changes it produced, or that subjects themselves have returned to the frameworks of identity that preceded COVID-19.

What is perhaps alarming, then, in this restoration of pre-pandemic practices is that the learnings about interdependency have not helped to prompt more equitable approaches, and have not transformed our practices of identity into ones oriented towards the universal grievability of all lives. Rather, many of the inequalities that made some lives more precarious (or lost) than others remain on the whole intact and in some cases have worsened. Rosi Braidotti (2020) identified the 'massive social inequalities' caused by neoliberal political classes as revealed in the 'horrid truth about the consequences of their austerity policies ... [and] the greed of consumers' society'. It is not that these inequities have been revealed and therefore should be the subject of policy, but that in the greater learning of our constitutional interdependency we are obliged to critically address these. Not because that will make populations more resilient during the next dangerous wave of COVID-19 or the next pandemic that may come, but because there is an ethical obligation at the heart of our constitution in interdependency that obliges us to recognize that all lives must be treated as equally grievable and to *prepare the social, health and caring infrastructure for that equality.*

To invoke infrastructure here is key, because we are not just interdependent with other human beings but with an ecology that provides that space, infrastructural supports and array of biological and social life that enables sustainability and survival. In invoking an ecology, it is important of course to be careful not to posit it as a pre-discursive 'nature' that due to some mystic property stabilizes bodies according to some notion of biology. An ecology, in Margaret Mead's (2017: 148–9) framework, is usually thought of as 'the mutual relations of organisms with their environment and with one another'. If bodies are interdependent from the beginning, then that is an interdependency constituted not only in the fact of that the interdependency precedes our subjectivity, but the fact that the interdependency occurs in a space of cohabitation, but within, through and emplaced by the conceptual and social ecologies that guarantee (for some) liveability, diversity and change. To incorporate a concept of ecology in this ethics is to recognize the significance of infrastructural support as a means by which interdependency can be more egalitarian and cohabitation sustained. This is a gamble, as it takes the focus away from the vulnerable body as the site of ethics, but a necessary one, since in our liberal-humanist culture the reference to corporeal subjectivity is always over-written by conceptual frames that violently differentiate and radically individuate bodies in ways that produce corporeal inequalities.

However, it is an important gamble, since it requires us to do two things: firstly, to consider the way in which a health infrastructure is not merely an institutional tool of caring (for some) but an integral part of the fabric of interdependent subjectivity that must be protected – even if protecting it means sometimes experiencing lockdowns to reduce its burden during times of need. Secondly, it means acknowledging that the ecology is not merely a setting for human life to flourish but that an interdependency is grounded in our shared cohabitation with other life, bringing both risk (such as the risk of incursion into places where new viruses jump species) and responsibility (such as extending practices of mutual care to a planet currently assaulted by carbon pollution resulting in substantial climate change). A learning from COVID that needs to be better incorporated into our social identities, forms of belonging and practices of relationality is one which is interdependent with the spaces in which interdependency occurs. And that obliges new, critical approaches to care.

Conclusion: Identity transformation

As I have argued throughout the chapters in this book, if our identities are performative and constituted in discourse, culture and sociality, then the disruption of the pandemic has to have re-constituted our identities differently, no matter how much the process of identity coherence calls on us to disavow or obscure that change. Some of the most important practices and ways of speaking about the pandemic were temporary whether the forms of health information and disinformation, the utilization of apocalyptic thinking, the immobilities of lockdowns, the deployment of mask-wearing or the social distancing calling upon people to avoid touch, and so on. Yet even in those uneven temporal phases, the cultural rupture of crisis experienced with suddenness and changed everydayness demands that performativity of subjectivity, identity and selfhood shifts substantially across the pandemic. At the time of writing, the pandemic has been with us for over three years, and with waning news coverage despite high rates of infection and continuing mortality, it is difficult to claim that there is a continuing culture of crisis. Nevertheless, for some that crisis continues in ways which impinge upon identity. I am thinking here particularly of those who now live with what is called 'long COVID' – the physical impact of having been infected that leaves some bodies infirm and incapable over a longer period, and which is experienced in diverse ways. Here, COVID is not something which is normalized but leaves some people with a loss of physicality that disrupts a sense of futurity not only at the cultural level but also in terms of other ways of experience an individual unknowability of the future and when – or if – those subjects will be well enough to experience full sociality again.

Attempting to calculate whether or not the shifts of health crisis are productive, beneficial, health, anxiety-provoking, major, minor or otherwise is not helpful at this stage, for such calculations always insist on producing new norms that thereby inculcate new marginalizations. Rather, what we might be optimistic about is that even in the face of some of the worst behaviour witnessed socially in many decades – rampant disinformation, refusal to participate, violent aggression, sovereign decisions that let some live and others die, the exacerbation of inequalities – the experience of disruption may have increased the sense of interdependency in such a way as to call for a better sociality based on equality of subjectivity and grievability for all, whether that all incorporates human populations or the wider ecology.

References

9News (2017), 'Majority of Australians Favour Public Burqa Ban according to New Poll', *9News*, 25 August. Available online: https://www.9news.com.au/national/majority-of-australians-favour-public-burqa-ban-according-to-new-poll/00bf7540-0a9e-4be2-a498-4828dd418aca (accessed 19 September 2022).

Abdelgadir, A. and V. Fouka (2020), 'Political Secularism and Muslim Integration in the West: Assessing the Effects of the French Headscarf Ban', *American Political Science Review*, 114 (3): 707–23.

ACL (2021), *Ask Your Leaders to Fully Restore Freedoms*, 28 August. Available online: https://www.acl.org.au/cm_nat_fearnot?fbclid=IwAR2AMep_riKzpmwkiqhTEr35AONHmsglmFG_8UFciaqLyzPdfrAuKEGPh1Y#splash-signup (accessed 28 August 2021).

Ahmed, S. (1999), 'Home and Away: Narratives of Migration and Estrangement', *International Journal of Cultural Studies*, 2 (3): 329–47.

Ahmed, S. (2004), *The Cultural Politics of Emotion*, Edinburgh: Edinburgh University Press.

Allcott, H. and M. Gentzkow (2017), 'Social Media and Fake News in the 2016 Election', *Journal of Economic Perspectives*, 31 (2): 211–36.

Andersen, K. G., A. Rambaut, W. I. Lipkin, E. C. Holmes and R. Garry (2020), 'The Proximal Origin of SARS-CoV-2', *Nature Medicine*, 26 (April): 450–2.

Anselmi, M. (2018), *Populism: An Introduction*, Abingdon & New York: Routledge.

Appadurai, A. (2003), 'Archive and Aspiration', in J. Brouwer and A. Mulder (eds), *Information Is Alive*, 14–25, Rotterdam: V2_Publishing and NAI Publishers.

Appadurai, A. (2004), 'The Capacity to Aspire: Culture and the Terms of Recognition', in V. Rao and M. Walton (eds), *Culture and Public Action*, 59–84, Stanford, CA: Stanford University Press.

Attwell, K., A. Hannah and J. Leask (2022), 'COVID-19: Talk of "Vaccine Hesitancy" Lets Governments off the Hook', *Nature*, 22 February. Available online: https://www.nature.com/articles/d41586-022-00495-8 (accessed 9 July 2022).

Attwell, K., J. K. Ward and S. Tomkinson (2021), 'Manufacturing Consent for Vaccine Mandates: A Comparative Case Study of Communication Campaigns in France and Australia', *Frontiers in Communication*, 23 February. Available online: https://doi.org/10.3389/fcomm.2021.598602 (accessed 19 October 2022).

Aubrey, S. (2020), 'He's Been Wearing a Mask for 30 Years. This Is What He Wants You to Know', *Sydney Morning Herald*, 26 July. Available online: https://www.smh.com.

au/lifestyle/life-and-relationships/he-s-been-wearing-a-mask-for-30-years-this-is-what-he-wants-you-to-know-20200722-p55eic.html (accessed 27 July 2020).

Aubusson, K. and M. Cunningham (2020), 'Virus Emergency Blueprint: Australia Pulls Trigger on Pandemic Plan', *Sydney Morning Herald*, 26 February. Available online: https://www.smh.com.au/national/virus-emergency-blueprint-australia-pulls-trigger-on-pandemic-plan-20200225-p54490.html (accessed 14 June 2020).

Bakhtin, M. (1984), *Rabelais and His World*, trans. H. Iswolsky, Bloomington, IN: Indiana University Press.

Barber, J. G. (2001), 'Relative Misery and Youth Suicide', *Australian and New Zealand Journal of Psychiatry*, 35 (1): 49–57.

Bartlett, A., K. Clarke and R. Cover (2019), *Flirting in the Era of #MeToo: Negotiating Intimacy*, Basingstoke: Palgrave Macmillan.

Battin, M. P. (1995), *Ethical Issues in Suicide*, Englewood Cliffs, NJ: Prentice-Hall.

BBC (2017), 'How Princess Diana Changed Attitudes to AIDS', *BBC News*, 5 April. Available online: https://www.bbc.com/news/av/magazine-39490507 (accessed 19 September 2022).

BBC (2020), 'Coronavirus Lockdown Protest: What's behind the US Demonstrations?', *BBC News*, 21 April. Available online: https://www.bbc.com/news/world-us-canada-52359100 (accessed 12 August 2022).

Beasley, C. (2008), 'Rethinking Hegemonic Masculinity in a Globalizing World', *Men and Masculinities*, 11 (1): 86–103.

Beck, A. T., A. Weissman, L. Trexler and D. Lester (1974), 'The Measurement of Pessimism: The Hopelessness Scale', *Journal of Consulting and Clinical Psychology*, 42 (6): 861–5.

Beck, U. (1998), *World Risk Society*, Cambridge: Polity Press.

Behind the News (2020), 'COVID Normal: What Does It Mean?', *YouTube*, 28 October. Available online: https://www.youtube.com/watch?v=v7GTQZ4JbSQ&ab_channel=BehindtheNews (accessed 19 September 2022).

Bell, V. (2010), 'New Scenes of Vulnerability, Agency and Plurality: An Interview with Judith Butler', *Theory, Culture & Society*, 27 (1): 130–52.

Bella, T. (2020), '"If I Get Corona, I Get Corona": Miami Spring Breakers Say Covid-19 hasn't Stopped Them from Partying', *Washington Post*, 19 March. Available online: https://www.washingtonpost.com/nation/2020/03/19/coronavirus-spring-break-party/ (accessed 12 September 2022).

Benn, S. I. (1982), 'Individuality, Autonomy and Community', in E. Kamenka (ed.), *Community as a Social Ideal*, 43–62, London: Edward Arnold.

Bennett, R. and K. Backholer (2021), *Online Food Delivery Is Surging during COVID-19 – But what are the Implications for Our Health?* Available online: https://iht.deakin.edu.au/2021/09/online-food-delivery-is-surging-during-covid-19-but-what-are-the-implications-for-our-health/ (accessed 12 September 2022).

Berger, E. (2021), 'More Children are Self-harming since the Start of the Pandemic', *The Conversation*, 8 September. Available online: https://theconversation.com/more-children-are-self-harming-since-the-start-of-the-pandemic-heres-what-parents-and-teachers-can-do-to-help-167436 (accessed 12 October 2022).

Berlant, L. (2007), 'Slow Death (Sovereignty, Obesity, Lateral Agency)', *Critical Inquiry*, 33 (4): 754–80.

Berlant, L. (2016), 'The Commons: Infrastructures for Troubling Times', *Environment and Planning D: Society & Space*, 34 (3): 393–419.

Bhabha, H. K. (1994), *The Location of Culture*, London and New York: Routledge.

Black, E. (2020), 'Daniel Andrews Rules out Sole Trader Exceptions, after Jim's Mowing Boss Calls for His Resignation', *SmartCompany*, 11 August. Available online: https://www.smartcompany.com.au/coronavirus/daniel-andrews-jims-mowing-boss-sole-trader-exceptions/ (accessed 18 September 2022).

Booker, C. (2021), 'Homeless Shown Hotel Door Between Lockdowns', *The Age*, 19 August. Available online: https://www.theage.com.au/national/victoria/homeless-being-turfed-from-hotels-during-lockdowns-lulls-20210819-p58k1i.html (accessed 19 August 2021).

Borger, J. (2020), 'White House Says "Business as Usual" as Trump Plays Down Coronavirus Threat', *The Guardian*, 10 March. Available online: https://www.theguardian.com/world/2020/mar/09/trump-coronavirus-white-house-response (accessed 13 August 2022).

Bowles, N. (2020), 'How to Prepare Now for the Complete End of the World', *New York Times*, 5 March. Available online: https://www.nytimes.com/2020/03/05/style/rewilding-stone-age-bushcraft.html%203/7 (accessed 16 March 2020).

Braidotti, R. (2020), '"We" Are in This Together, but We Are Not One and the Same', *Journal of Bioethical Inquiry*, 17 (4): 465–9.

Breakey, H. (2021), 'Public Protest or Selfish Ratbaggery? Why Free Speech Doesn't Give You the Right to Endanger Other People's Health', *The Conversation*, 27 July. Available online: https://theconversation.com/public-protest-or-selfish-ratbaggery-why-free-speech-doesnt-give-you-the-right-to-endanger-other-peoples-health-165079 (accessed 21 September 2022).

Brennan, J. (2018), 'A Libertarian Case for Mandatory Vaccination', *Journal of Medical Ethics*, 44 (1): 37–43.

Brown, A. L. (2022), 'Italy Eliminates Sanctions against Anti-Vaccine Health Personnel', *Prensa Latina*, 28 October. Available online: https://www.plenglish.com/news/2022/10/28/italy-eliminates-sanctions-against-anti-vaccine-health-personnel/ (accessed 29 October 2022).

Brown, H. and A. M. Sáez (2021), 'Ebola Separations: Trust, Crisis, and "Social Distancing" in West Africa', *The Journal of the Royal Anthropological Institute*, 27 (1): 9–29.

Brugère, F. (2019), *Care Ethics: The Introduction of Care as Political Category*, trans. A. Chrétien, O. Cooper-Hadjian and B. Heffernan, Leuven: Peeters Publishers.

Bruns, A. (2019), *Are Filter Bubbles Real?* London: Polity.

Buhler, B. (2020), 'How COVID-19 Has Brought Delivery into the Future', *Accenture*, 28 July. Available online: https://www.accenture.com/au-en/blogs/voices-public-service/how-covid-19-has-brought-delivery-into-the-future (accessed 19 September 2022).

Burgess, J. and J. Green (2009), *YouTube: Online Video and Participatory Culture*, Cambridge: Polity.

Butler, J. (1990), *Gender Trouble: Feminism and the Subversion of Identity*, London: Routledge.

Butler, J. (1991), 'Imitation and Gender Insubordination', in D. Fuss (ed.), *Inside/Out: Lesbian Theories, Gay Theories*, 13–31, London: Routledge.

Butler, J. (1993), *Bodies That Matter: On the Discursive Limits of 'Sex'*, London & New York: Routledge.

Butler, J. (1997), *The Psychic Life of Power: Theories in Subjection*, Stanford, CA: Stanford University Press.

Butler, J. (2003), 'Violence, Mourning, Politics', *Studies in Gender and Sexuality*, 4 (1): 9–37.

Butler, J. (2004), *Precarious Life*, London: Verso.

Butler, J. (2006), 'The Desire to Live: Spinoza's Ethics under Pressure', in V. Kahn, N. Saccamano and D. Coli (eds), *Politics and the Passions 1500–1850*, 111–30, Princeton, NJ: Princeton University Press.

Butler, J. (2009), *Frames of War: When Is Life Grievable?* London & New York: Verso.

Butler, J. (2012), *Parting Ways: Jewishness and the Critique of Zionism*, New York: Columbia University Press.

Butler, J. (2015), *Notes toward a Performative Theory of Assembly*, Cambridge, MA: Harvard University Press.

Butler, J. (2020), *The Force of Nonviolence: An Ethico-Political Bind*, London: Verso.

Butler, J. and A. Athanasiou (2013), *Dispossession: The Performative in the Political*, Cambridge: Polity.

Butler, J. and G. C. Spivak (2007), *Who Sings the Nation-State? Language, Politics, Belonging*, London: Seagull Books.

Cadesky, E. (2020), 'Coronavirus and Cognitive Bias: The Surprising Reasons People Cheat at Social Distancing', *The Conversation*, 21 May. Available online: https://theconversation.com/coronavirus-and-cognitive-bias-the-surprising-reasons-people-cheat-at-social-distancing-137987 (accessed 22 September 2022).

Califia, P. (1994), *Public Sex: The Culture of Radical Sex*, Pittsburgh: Cleis Press.

Caputo, J. D. (1993), *Against Ethics: Contributions to a Poetics of Obligation with Constant Reference to Deconstruction*, Bloomington, IN: Indiana University Press.

Carballo-Carbajal, I. (2021), 'Flawed Speculative Study Incorrectly Claims That mRNA COVID-19 Vaccines Cause Neurodegenerative Diseases', *Health Feedback*, 29 April. Available online: https://healthfeedback.org/claimreview/flawed-speculative-study-incorrectly-claims-that-mrna-covid-19-vaccines-cause-neurodegenerative-diseases/ (accessed 3 September 2022).

Carey, J. (1988), *Communication as Culture: Essays on Media and Society*, London: Routledge.

Caruth, C. (1995), 'Recapturing the Past', in C. Caruth (ed.), *Trauma: Explorations in Memory*, 151–7, Baltimore: Johns Hopkins University Press.

Castells, M. (2000), *The Rise of the Network Society*, Oxford: Blackwell.

Cathey, L. (2020), 'Fact Checking Trump's Claim about Suicides if the Economic Shutdown Continues', *ABC News*, 26 March. Available online: https://abcnews. go.com/Politics/fact-checking-trumps-claim-suicide-thousands-economic-shutdown/story?id=69790273 (accessed 20 September 2022).

Centers for Disease Control and Prevention (2011), *A CDC Framework for Preventing Infectious Diseases: Sustaining the Essentials and Innovating for the Future*, October. Available online: https://www.cdc.gov/oid/docs/ID-Framework.pdf (accessed 12 July 2022).

Centers for Disease Control and Prevention (2022), *Coughing and Sneezing*, 15 June. Available online: https://www.cdc.gov/hygiene/personal-hygiene/coughing-sneezing.html (accessed 5 October 2022).

Chapman, E. (2000), 'Conceptualisation of the Body for People Living with HIV: Issues of Touch and Contamination', *Sociology of Health & Illness*, 22 (6): 840–857.

Chrisoulakis, N. (2021), 'The Part of Your Body That Will Help Most with Pandemic Stress', *The Age*, 22 August. Available online: https://www.theage.com.au/lifestyle/ health-and-wellness/the-part-of-your-body-that-will-help-most-with-pandemic-stress-20210819-p58k42.html (accessed 22 August 2021).

Christie, A. and H. Mittler (1999), 'Partnership and Core Groups in the Risk Society', *Child and Family Social Work*, 4 (3): 231–40.

Clough, P. T. (2008), 'The Affective Turn: Political Economy, Biomedia and Bodies', *Theory, Culture & Society*, 25 (1): 1–22.

Clun, R. (2020), ' "Skipped a Decade": Tele-health to Become Permanent after Success during Pandemic', *Sydney Morning Herald*, 27 November. Available online: https:// www.smh.com.au/politics/federal/skipped-a-decade-tele-health-to-become-permanent-after-success-during-pandemic-20201127-p56ik0.html (accessed 30 February 2021).

Clun, R. (2021), 'Fewer Suicides, but Alcohol-Related Deaths Rose in First Pandemic Year', *Sydney Morning Herald*, 29 September. Available online: https://www.smh. com.au/politics/federal/fewer-suicides-but-alcohol-related-deaths-rose-in-first-pandemic-year-20210929-p58vpn.html (accessed 30 September 2021).

Cole, K. A. (2004), '"Men in White" on Television: An Exercise in Cultural Power', in L. D. Friedman (ed.), *Cultural Sutures: Medicine and Media*, 93–108, Durham, NC: Duke University Press.

Connell, R. W. (1995), *Masculinities*, Cambridge: Polity.

Connolly, W. E. (1991), *Identity/Difference: Democratic Negotiations of Political Paradox*, Ithaca, NY: Cornell University Press.

Cooper, S. (2000), *Relating to Queer Theory: Rereading Sexual Self-Definition with Irigaray, Kristeva, Wittig and Cixous*, Bern: Peter Lang.

Council of the European Union (2022), *Member States Agree on a Temporary Waiver from Slot Rules at EU Airports*, 12 October. Available online: https://www.consilium. europa.eu/en/press/press-releases/2022/10/12/member-states-agree-on-a-temporary-waiver-from-slot-rules-at-eu-airports/ (accessed 29 October 2022).

Cover, R. (2006), 'Audience Inter/active: Interactive Media, Narrative Control and Reconceiving Audience History', *New Media & Society*, 8 (1): 213–32.

Cover, R. (2013a), 'Undoing Attitudes: Ethical Change in the Go Back to Where You Came From Documentary', *Continuum: Journal of Media & Cultural Studies*, 27 (3): 408–20.

Cover, R. (2013b), 'Suspended Ethics and the Team: Theorising Sportsplayers' Group Sexual Assault in the Context of Identity', *Sexualities*, 16 (3–4): 300–18.

Cover, R. (2015), 'Mobility, Belonging and Bodies: Understanding Attitudes of Anxiety towards Temporary Migrants in Australia', *Continuum: Journal of Media & Cultural Studies*, 29 (1): 32–44.

Cover, R. (2016), *Digital Identities: Creating and Communicating the Online Self*, London: Elsevier.

Cover, R. (2019), *Emergent Identities: New Sexualities, Gender and Relationships in a Digital Era*, London & New York: Routledge.

Cover, R. (2020a), *Population, Mobility and Belonging: Understanding Population Concepts in Media, Culture and Society*, London & New York: Routledge.

Cover, R. (2020b), 'Vulnerability and the Discourse of "Forgotten People": Populism, Population and Cultural Change', *Continuum: Journal of Media & Cultural Studies*, 34 (5): 749–62.

Cover, R. (2020c), 'Subjective Connectivity: Rethinking Loneliness, Isolation and Belonging in Discourses of Minority Youth Suicide', *Social Epistemology*, 34 (6): 566–76.

Cover, R. (2022), 'Digital Hostility: Contemporary Crisis, Disrupted Belonging and Self-Care Practices', *Media International Australia*, 184 (1): 79–91.

Cover, R., A. Haw and J. D. Thompson (2022), *Fake News in Digital Cultures: Technology, Populism and Digital Misinformation*, London: Emerald.

Creed, B. (2003), *Media Matrix: Sexing the New Reality*, St. Leonards, NSW: Allen & Unwin.

Cunningham, M. (2022), '"A Dire Situation That Is Unprecedented": Senior Alfred Doctor Quits, Warning of Mass Burnout', *The Age*, 12 May. Available online: https:// www.theage.com.au/national/victoria/a-dire-situation-that-is-unprecedented-

senior-alfred-doctor-quits-warning-of-mass-burnout-20220511-p5akcx.
html#:~:text=A%20senior%20doctor%20at%20Melbourne's,healthcare%20
workers%20to%20breaking%20point (accessed 13 May 2022).

Daddow, O. (2013), 'Margaret Thatcher, Tony Blair and the Eurosceptic Tradition in
Britain', *The British Journal of Politics and International Relations*, 15 (2): 210–27.

de Certeau, M. (1984), *The Practice of Everyday Life*, Berkeley, CA: University of
California Press.

Depoux, A., S. Martin, E. Karafillakis, R. Preet, A. Wilder-Smith and H. Larson (2020),
'The Pandemic of Social Media Panic Travels Faster than the COVID-19 Outbreak',
Journal of Travel Medicine, 27 (3): 1–2.

Derrida, J. (1978), *Writing and Difference*, trans. A. Bass. Chicago: University of
Chicago Press.

Derrida, J. (1999), *Adieu to Emmanuel Levinas*, trans. P. A Brault and M. Naas, Stanford,
CA: Stanford University Press.

Derrida, J. (2001), *On Cosmopolitanism and Forgiveness*, trans. M. Dooley and M.
Hughes. London: Routledge.

Dewey, C. (2016), 'Facebook Fake-News Writer: "I Think Donald Trump Is in the White
House because of Me', *Washington Post*, 17 November. Available online : https://
www.washingtonpost.com/news/the-intersect/wp/2016/11/17/facebook-fake-
news-writer-i-think-donald-trump-is-in-the-white-house-because-of-me/?utm_
term=.42ceafd555c6 (accessed 12 December 2016).

Dexter, R. and E. Pearson (2020), 'Thousands Flock to St Kilda Beach, Many Maskless,
as Hot Weather Hits', *The Age*, 3 November. Available online: https://www.theage.
com.au/national/victoria/thousands-flock-to-st-kilda-beach-many-maskless-as-hot-
weather-hits-20201103-p56b85.html (accessed 4 November 2020).

Douglas, K. M., J. E. Uscinski, R. M. Sutton, A. Cichocka, T. Nefes, C. S. Ang and F.
Deravi (2019), 'Understanding Conspiracy Theories', *Political Psychology*, 40 (3–5):
3–35.

Downer, J. and M. Kekewich (2021), 'Improving Family Access to Dying Patients
during the COVID-19 Pandemic', *The Lancet*, 12 January. Available online: https://
doi.org/10.1016/S2213-2600(21)00025-4 (accessed 12 October 2022).

Dreher, T. (2009), 'Listening across Difference: Media and Multiculturalism beyond
the Politics of Voice', *Continuum: Journal of Media & Cultural Studies*, 23 (4):
445–58.

Duggan, L. (2003), *The Twilight of Equality? Neoliberalism, Cultural Politics and the
Attack on Democracy*, Boston, MA: Beacon Press.

Durkheim, E. (1952), *Suicide: A Study in Sociology*, trans. J. A. Spaulding and G.
Simpson, London: Routledge & Kegan Paul.

Ehrlich, P. R. (1968), *The Population Bomb*, New York: Ballantine.

Evers, C. (2008), 'The Cronulla Race Riots: Safety Maps on an Australian Beach', *South
Atlantic Quarterly*, 107 (2): 411–29.

Faine, J. (2021), 'Use COVID-19 to Bring People Together, Not Push Them Apart', *The Age*, 15 August. Available online: https://www.theage.com.au/national/use-covid-19-to-bring-people-together-not-push-them-apart-20210813-p58igs.html (accessed 19 August 2022).

Faist, T. (2013), 'The Mobility Turn: A New Paradigm for the Social Sciences?', *Ethnic and Racial Studies*, 36 (11): 1637–46.

Featherstone, M. (2006), 'Archive', *Theory, Culture & Society*, 23 (2–3): 591–6.

Fisher, M. (2020), 'Flushing out the True Cause of the Global Toilet Paper Shortage Amid Coronavirus Pandemic', *The Washington Post*, 7 April. Available online: https://www.washingtonpost.com/national/coronavirus-toilet-paper-shortage-panic/2020/04/07/1fd30e92-75b5-11ea-87da-77a8136c1a6d_story.html (accessed 12 April 2020).

Fiske, J. (1989), *Understanding Popular Culture*, London: Unwin Hyman.

Fitzsimmons, C. and D. Snow (2020), 'Catalyst for Change: How the Pandemic Changed the Way We Live and Work', *The Age*, 13 December. Available online: https://www.theage.com.au/politics/federal/catalyst-for-change-how-the-pandemic-changed-the-way-we-live-and-work-20201203-p56k8b.html (accessed 13 December 2020).

Flew, T. (2008), *New Media: An Introduction*, third edition, Melbourne: Oxford University Press.

Forrest, J., K. Blair and K. Dunn (2020), 'Racist Attitudes, Out-Groups and the Australian Experience', *Australian Journal of Social Issues*, 56 (1): 78–93.

Forsey, Z. (2020), 'Woman with Coronavirus Explains What It's Really Like – with Chilling Warning', *Mirror*, 12 March. Available online: https://www.mirror.co.uk/news/world-news/woman-coronavirus-explains-what-its-21680170 (accessed 18 August 2022).

Foucault, M. (1973), *The Birth of the Clinic: An Archaeology of Medical Perception*, trans. A. M. Sheridan Smith, New York: Pantheon.

Foucault, M. (1977), *Discipline and Punish: The Birth of the Prison*, trans. A. Sheridan, London: Penguin.

Foucault, M. (2004a), *Society Must Be Defended: Lectures at the Collège de France, 1975–76*, ed. M. Bvertani and A. Fontana, trans. D. Macey, London: Penguin.

Foucault, M. (2004b), *Abnormal: Lectures at the Collège de France 1974–1975*, ed. V. Marchetti and A. Salmoni, trans. G. Burchell, New York: Picador.

Foucault, M. (2005), *The Hermeneutics of the Subject: Lectures at the Collège de France, 1981–82*, ed. F. Gros, trans. G. Burchell, New York: Picador.

Foucault, M. (2007), *Security, Territory, Population: Lectures at the Collège de France, 1977–78*, trans. G. Burchell, ed. M. Senellart, Hampshire: Palgrave Macmillan.

Foucault, M. (2008), *The Birth of Biopolitics: Lectures at the Collège de France, 1978–79*, ed. M. Senellart, trans. G. Burchell, Hampshire: Palgrave Macmillan.

Freelon, D. and C. Wells (2020), 'Disinformation as Political Communication', *Political Communication*, 37 (2): 145–56.

Freeman, E. (2010), *Time Binds: Queer Temporalities, Queer Histories*, Durham, NC: Duke University Press.

Freud, S. (1994), 'Mourning and Melancholia' [1917], in *The Standard Edition of the Complete Psychological Works of Sigmund Freud*, J. Strachey (trans.), volume XIV, 243–58, London: Hogarth.

Fukuyama, F. (2019), *Identity: Contemporary Identity Politics and the Struggle for Recognition*, London: Profile Books.

Fuss, D. (1995), *Identification Papers*, New York & London: Routledge.

Gilson, E. (2011), 'Vulnerability, Ignorance, and Oppression', *Hypatia*, 26 (2): 308–32.

Godlee, F., J. Smith and H. Marcovitch (2011), 'Wakefield's Article Linking MMR Vaccine and Autism was Fraudulent', *BMJ*, 19 (1): 8.

Goldsmith, A. (2020), 'How 10 Fictional Pandemics Compare to Ours, from Contagion's MEV-1 to Outbreak's Motaba', *Town & Country*, 13 May. Available online: https://www.townandcountrymag.com/leisure/arts-and-culture/g32419194/pandemic-movies/ (accessed 20 July 2020).

Grab, A. (2015), 'The Napoleonic State and Public Health Policies: Smallpox Vaccination in Napoleonic Italy (1800–1814)', *Società e Storia* (January): 487–511. Available online: http://doi.10.3280/SS2014-145003 (accessed 13 July 2022).

Gramsci, A. (1971), *Selections from the Prison Notebooks of Antonio Gramsci*, ed. and trans. Q. Hoare and G. N. Smith, London: Lawrence & Wishart.

Great Barrington Declaration (2020), *Great Barrington Declaration*, 4 October. Available online: https://gbdeclaration.org/ (accessed 19 September 2022).

Grisar, P. J. (2020), 'What Does the Bible Say about Quarantine?', *Forward*, 9 March. Available online: https://forward.com/culture/441195/what-does-the-bible-say-about-quarantine/ (accessed 18 September 2022).

Groch, S. (2020), 'Speckled Monsters and Graverobbers: What Can We Learn from the Killer Plagues of History?', *The Age*, 26 April. Available online: https://www.theage.com.au/national/speckled-monsters-and-graverobbers-how-did-past-pandemics-end-and-how-does-this-one-compare-20200415-p54k31.html (accessed 21 May 2020).

Grosz, E. (1995), *Space, Time and Perversion: The Politics of Bodies*, London: Routledge.

Hall, B. and R. Dexter (2021), 'Generation COVID-19: Are the Kids Going to Be All Right?' *The Age*, 23 October. Available online: https://www.theage.com.au/national/victoria/generation-covid-19-are-the-kids-going-to-be-all-right-20211020-p591p7.html (accessed 12 September 2022).

Hall, S. (1979), 'The Great Moving Right Show', *Marxism Today* (January): 14–20.

Hall, S. (1993), 'Encoding/Decoding', in S. During (ed.), *The Cultural Studies Reader*, 90–103, London: Routledge.

Hall, S. (1995), 'The Whites of Their Eyes: Racist Ideologies and the Media', in G. Dines and J. M. Humez (eds), *Gender, Race and Class in Media: A Text-Reader*, 18–22, Thousand Oaks, CA: Sage.

Harvey, J. (2021), 'Doctor Laughs Out Loud at Tinfoil Hat-Worthy Suspicion about Vaccines', *HuffPost*, 3 May. Available online: https://www.huffpost.com/entry/coronavirus-vaccine-tracking-devices_n_608a3633e4b0ccb91c2dd0e2 (accessed 12 September 2022).

Harvey, R. (2012), 'Young People, Sexual Orientation, and Resilience', in M. Unger (ed.), *The Social Ecology of Resilience: A Handbook of Theory and Practice*, 325–35, New York: Springer.

Hickey-Moody, A. (2016), 'Youth Agency and Adult Influence: A Critical Revision of Little Publics', *Review of Education, Pedagogy, and Cultural Studies*, 38 (1): 58–72.

Holden, R. R, J. C. Mendonca and R. C. Serin (1989), 'Suicide, Hopelessness, and Social Desirability: A Test of an Interactive Model', *Journal of Consulting and Clinical Psychology*, 57 (4): 500–4.

Holling, C. S. (1973), 'Resilience and Stability of Ecological Systems', *Annual Review of Ecology and Systematics*, 4 (1): 1–23.

Horlick-Jones, T. (2003), 'Commentary: Managing Risk and Contingency: Interaction and Accounting Behaviour', *Health, Risk & Society*, 5 (2): 221–8.

Horlick-Jones, T. (2005), '"On 'Risk Work": Professional Discourse, Accountability, and Everyday Action', *Health, Risk & Society*, 7 (3): 293–307.

Horowitz, J. (2020), "Italians Find 'a Moment of Joy in This Moment of Anxiety'", *New York Times*, 14 March. Available online: https://www.nytimes.com/2020/03/14/world/europe/italians-find-a-moment-of-joy-in-this-moment-of-anxiety.html (accessed 19 August 2022).

Hui, S. and G. Faulconbridge (2021), 'Partygoers Celebrate England's "Freedom Day" Amid Warnings of a Nasty Hangover', *The Age*, 19 July. Available online: https://www.theage.com.au/world/europe/nightclubs-elated-but-england-s-freedom-day-could-leave-a-nasty-hangover-20210718-p58asi.html (accessed 20 July 2021).

Huizinga, J. (1949), *Homo Ludens: A Study of the Play-Element in Culture*, London: Routledge & Kegan Paul.

Illingworth, G., K. L. Mansfield, C. A. Espie, M. Fazel and F. Waite (2022), 'Sleep in the Time of COVID-19: Findings from 17000 School-Aged Children and Adolescents in the UK during the First National Lockdown', *Sleep Advances*, 3 (1): zpab021.

Inglehart, R. F. and P. Morris (2016), 'Trump, Brexit, and the Rise of Populism: Economic Have-Nots and Cultural Backlash', *Harvard Kennedy School Working Paper Series*, Number 26. Available online: https://papers.ssrn.com/sol3/papers.cfm?abstract_id=2818659 (accessed 9 January 2021).

Jackall, R. (1995), *Propaganda*, Basingstoke: Macmillan.

Jackson, A. (2020), 'Our Social Safety Net Faces Its Biggest Test in Generations', *The Age*, 29 March. Available online: https://www.theage.com.au/national/our-social-safety-net-faces-its-biggest-test-in-generations-20200329-p54eyt.html (accessed 13 November 2021).

Jenkins, S. (2020), 'Why I'm Taking the Coronavirus Hype with a Pinch of Salt', *The Guardian*, 7 March. Available online: https://www.theguardian.com/commentisfree/2020/mar/06/coronavirus-hype-crisis-predictions-sars-swine-flu-panics (accessed 12 August 2022).

Jiang, J., X. Ren and E. Ferrara (2021), 'Social Media Polarization and Echo Chambers in the Context of COVID-19: Case Study', *JMIRx Med*, 2 (3): e29570.

Joiner, T. (2005), *Why People Die by Suicide*, Cambridge, MA: Harvard University Press.

Joyce, C. (2020), *Open Letter to Prime Minister from Concerned Australians on Need to Exit COVID-19 Lockdown*, 24 April. Available online: https://www.livewiremarkets.com/wires/open-letter-to-prime-minister-from-concerned-australians-on-need-to-exit-covid-19-lockdown (accessed 11 April 2021).

Kendall-Tackett, K. A. (2017), *Depression in New Mothers: Causes, Consequences, and Treatment Alternatives*, third edition, London and New York: Routledge.

Knaus, C. (2022), ' "Avi Out": The Uncomfortable Relationship between Rebel News and Australia's Anti-Vaccine Protesters', *The Guardian*, 11 February. Available online: https://www.theguardian.com/australia-news/2022/feb/11/avi-out-the-uncomfortable-relationship-between-rebel-news-and-australias-anti-vaccine-protesters (accessed 22 September 2022).

Knott, M. (2021a), ' "Workers Are Empowered": The Four Factors Driving America's "Great Resignation"', *The Age*, 13 November. Available online: https://www.theage.com.au/world/north-america/workers-are-empowered-the-four-factors-driving-america-s-great-resignation-20211113-p598l7.html (accessed 13 November 2021).

Knott, M. (2021b), 'Fringe, Feasible or False? The COVID-19 Wuhan Lab Leak Theory Gets a Second Look', *Sydney Morning Herald*, 23 May. Available online: https://www.smh.com.au/world/north-america/fringe-feasible-or-false-the-covid-19-wuhan-lab-leak-theory-gets-a-second-look-20210521-p57tts.html (accessed 12 September 2022).

Kokkegård, H. (2022), 'Social Media Echo Chambers Spread Vaccine Misinformation', *DTU*, 16 February. Available online: https://www.dtu.dk/english/news/all-news/nyhed?id=185ae340-3cab-4709-95b3-a9548ad51580 (accessed 19 September 2022).

Koob, S. F. and C. Butt (2020), 'Hundreds of Thousands Call Police to Dob in Coronavirus Breaches', *The Age*, 3 October. Available online: https://www.theage.com.au/national/victoria/hundreds-of-thousands-call-police-to-dob-in-coronavirus-breaches-20201002-p561ij.html (accessed 6 October 2020).

Kral, M. J. (1994), 'Suicide as Social Logic', *Suicide & Life-Threatening Behavior*, 24 (3): 245–59.

Kristeva, J. (1982), *Powers of Horror: An Essay on Abjection*, trans. L. S. Roudiez. New York: Columbia University Press.

Kuo, L., L. Li and V. Chiang P.-L. Wu (2022), 'Shanghai's Covid Siege: Food Shortages, Talking Robots, Starving Animals', *Washington Post*, 15 April. Available online: https://

www.washingtonpost.com/world/interactive/2022/china-shanghai-covid-lockdown-food-shortage/ (accessed 22 September 2022).

La Caze, M. (2011), 'Terrorism and Trauma: Negotiating Derridean "Autoimmunity"', *Philosophy & Social Criticism*, 37 (5): 605–19.

Lacina, L. (2020), 'Should You Wear a Face Mask? WHO Officials Weigh in at Today's COVID-19 Briefing', *World Economic Forum*, 30 March. Available online: https://www.weforum.org/agenda/2020/03/who-should-wear-a-face-mask-30-march-who-briefing/ (accessed 11 July 2022).

Lazzarato, M. (2011), *The Making of Indebted Man: An Essay on the Neoliberal Condition*, trans. J. D. Jordan, South Pasadena, CA: Semiotext(e).

Lazzarato, M. (2013), *Governing by Debt*, trans. J. D. Jordan, South Pasadena, CA: Semiotext(e).

Le Grand, C. (2022), 'Melbourne Ground Zero for Lockdown Harms, Says Health Expert', *The Age*, 24 September. Available online: https://www.theage.com.au/national/victoria/melbourne-ground-zero-for-lockdown-harms-says-health-expert-20220922-p5bkcc.html (accessed 24 September 2022).

Lee, B. Y. (2021), 'As Covid-19 Vaccine Microchip Conspiracy Theories Spread, Here Are Responses on Twitter', *Forbes*, 8 May. Available online: https://www.forbes.com/sites/brucelee/2021/05/09/as-covid-19-vaccine-microchip-conspiracy-theories-spread-here-are-some-responses/?sh=22736e41602d (accessed 9 August 2022).

Leipold, B. and W. Greve (2009), 'Resilience: A Conceptual Bridge between Coping and Development', *European Psychologist*, 14 (1): 40–50.

Lemke, T. (2011), *Bio-politics: An Advanced Introduction*, trans. E. F. Trump, New York: New York University Press.

Levinas, E. (1969), *Totality and Infinity*, trans. A. Lingis, Pittsburgh, PA: Duquesne University Press.

Lewis, D. (2022a), 'Why the WHO Took Two Years to Say COVID Is Airborne', *Nature*, 6 April. Available online: https://www.nature.com/articles/d41586-022-00925-7#:~:text=It%20took%20until%202020%20October,crowded%20and%20inadequately%20ventilated%20spaces (accessed 12 September 2022).

Lewis, D. (2022b), *Unvaxxed: Trust, Truth and the Rise of Vaccine Outrage*, Richmond, VIC and London: Hardie Grant Books.

Lewis, J. D. and A. Weigert (1985), 'Trust as a Social Reality', *Social Forces*, 63 (4): 967–85.

Lifeline (2020), *Media Release*, 22 December. Available online: https://www.lifeline.org.au/resources/news-and-media-releases/media-releases/ (accessed 28 August 2021).

Linderman, N. (2021), 'Report: Pfizer Vaccine Confirmed to Cause Neurodegenerative Diseases – Study', *National File*, 22 April. Available online: https://archive.ph/iRyaB#selection-935.0-938.0 (accessed 3 September 2022).

Lingis, A. (1994), *The Community of Those Who Have Nothing in Common*, Bloomington & Indianapolis, IN: Indiana University Press.

Locke, J. (1988), *Two Treatises of Government*, ed. P. Laslett, Cambridge: Cambridge University Press.

Lucas, C., M. Cunningham, N. Towell, E. Pearson, J. Topsfield and A. Prytz (2021), 'Fatigue Weighs Heavy as Victoria Snaps Back into Lockdown', *The Age*, 17 July. Available online: https://www.theage.com.au/politics/victoria/fatigue-weighs-heavy-as-melbourne-snaps-back-into-lockdown-20210714-p589t3.html (accessed 12 September 2022).

Lupton, D., C. Southerton, M. Clark and A. Watson (2021), *The Face Mask in COVID Times: A Sociomaterial Analysis*, Berlin: de Gruyter.

Lynteris, C. (2018), 'Plague Masks: The Visual Emergence of Anti-epidemic Personal Protection Equipment', *Medical Anthropology*, 37 (6): 442–57.

Ma, Y. and N. Zhan (2022), 'To Mask or Not to Mask amid the COVID-19 Pandemic: How Chinese Students in America Experience and Cope with Stigma', *Chinese Sociological Review*, 54 (1): 1–26.

Macey, D. (2009), 'Rethinking Biopolitics, Race and Power in the Wake of Foucault', *Theory, Culture & Society*, 26 (6): 186–205.

Maddox, G. (2020), '"I Need to Shut It Down Fast": How Our Leisure Activities Came to a Sudden Halt', *The Age*, 14 December. Available online: https://www.theage.com.au/national/i-need-to-shut-it-down-fast-how-our-leisure-activities-came-to-a-sudden-halt-20201119-p56g6a.html (accessed 20 December 2020).

Maguire, Danielle (2020), 'Coronavirus May Have Killed the Handshake, but Are Elbow Bumps Any Better?' *ABC News*, 19 March. Available online: https://www.abc.net.au/news/2020-03-17/coronavirus-killed-the-handshake-what-are-alternatives/12064176?nw=0 (accessed 14 July 2021).

Mair, S. (2020), 'What will the World Be Like after Coronavirus? Four Possible Futures', *The Conversation*, 30 March. Available online: https://theconversation.com/what-will-the-world-be-like-after-coronavirus-four-possible-futures-134085 (accessed 19 September 2022).

Mannell, K. and J. Meese (2022), 'From Doom-Scrolling to News Avoidance: Limiting News as a Wellbeing Strategy during COVID Lockdown', *Journalism Studies*, 23 (2): 302–19.

Mao, F. (2020), 'Coronavirus Panic: Why are People Stockpiling Toilet Paper?', *BBC News*, 4 March. Available online: https://www.bbc.com/news/world-australia-51731422 (accessed 18 August 2022).

Marcuse, H. (1964), *One Dimensional Man*, London: Abacus.

Matza, M. (2020), 'What Is the "Sovereign Citizen" Movement?', *BBC News*, 5 August. Available online: https://www.bbc.com/news/world-us-canada-53654318 (accessed 31 August 2022).

McCann, C. M, E. Beddoe, K. McCormick, P. Huggard, S. Kedge, C. Adamson and J. Huggard (2013), 'Resilience in the Health Professions: A Review of Recent Literature', *International Journal of Wellbeing*, 3 (1): 60–81.

McCoy, T. S. (1993), *Voices of Difference: Studies in Critical Philosophy and Mass Communication*, Cresskill, NJ: Hampton Press.

McGuiness, P. P. (2021), 'Want to Be Part of the Fashionable Set? Don't Join the "Freethinkers"', *The Age*, 19 June. Available online: https://www.theage.com.au/national/want-to-be-part-of-the-fashionable-set-don-t-join-the-freethinkers-20210618-p58270.html (accessed 19 June 2021).

McGuinness, P. (2021), 'A Long History and Iconic Moments: Will We Ever Shake Hands Again?', *The Age*, 27 August. Available online: https://www.theage.com.au/culture/books/put-it-there-but-will-we-ever-shake-again-20210819-p58k7q.html (accessed 9 September 2021).

McKee, A., K. Albury, J. Burgess, B. Light, K. Osman and A. Walsh (2018), 'Locked Down Apps versus the Social Media Ecology: Why Do Young People and Educators Disagree on the Best Delivery Platform for Digital Sexual Health Entertainment Education?', *New Media & Society*, 20 (12): 4571–4589.

McMillan, A. and K. Papworth (2020), 'Shoppers Empty Shelves as Virus Panic Takes Hold', *The Age*, 14 March. Available online: https://www.theage.com.au/national/victoria/sea-of-shoppers-empties-shelves-as-virus-panic-takes-hold-20200314-p54a1z.html (accessed 15 March 2020).

McNeill, W. H. (1976), *Plagues and Peoples*, New York: Anchor.

Mead, M. (2017), *Continuities in Cultural Evolution*, London & New York: Routledge.

Milan, S. (2020), 'Techno-Solutionism and the Standard Human in the Making of the COVID-19 Pandemic', *Big Data & Society*. Available online: https://doi.org/10.1177/2053951720966781 (accessed 12 September 2022).

Mill, J. S. (1972), *Utilitarianism, On Liberty, and Considerations on Representative Government*, ed. H. B. Acton. London: J. M. Dent & Sons.

Miller, C. (2020), 'Coronavirus: Far-right Spreads Covid-19 "Infodemic" on Facebook', *BBC News*, 4 May. Available online: https://www.bbc.com/news/technology-52490430 (accessed 5 May 2020).

Miller, J. M. (2020), 'Do COVID-19 Conspiracy Theory Beliefs Form a Monological Belief System?', *Canadian Journal of Political Science*, 53 (2): 319–26.

Milligan, S. (2020), 'Trump's Choice: The Economy or Human Lives', *U.S. News*, 24 March. Available online: https://www.usnews.com/news/national-news/articles/2020-03-24/trumps-choice-on-coronavirus-the-economy-or-human-lives (accessed 1 September 2022).

Mitchell, A. and J. B. Oliphant (2020), 'Americans Immersed in COVID-19 News: Most Think Media Are Doing Fairly Well Covering It', *Pew Research Center*. Available online: https://www.journalism.org/2020/03/18/americansimmersed-in-covid-19-news-most-think-media-are-doing-fairly-wellcovering-it/ (accessed 12 September 2022).

Moore, A. (2020), 'How the Coronavirus Created a Toilet Paper Shortage', *NC State University College of Natural Resources News*, 19 May. Available online: https://cnr.

ncsu.edu/news/2020/05/coronavirus-toilet-paper-shortage/ (accessed 18 August 2022).

Muecke, S. (2007), 'Hurricane Katrina and the Rhetoric of Natural Disasters', in E. Potter et al. (eds), *Fresh Water: New Perspectives on Water in Australia*, 259–72, Melbourne: Melbourne University Press.

Munt, S. (2002), 'Framing Intelligibility, Identity, and Selfhood: A Reconsideration of Spatio-Temporal Models', *Reconstruction*, 2 (3). Available online: http://www.reconstruction.ws/023/munt.htm (accessed 3 January 2003).

Munt, S. (2007), *Queer Attachments: The Cultural Politics of Shame*, Aldershot: Ashgate.

Nikolaidis, A. (2011), 'Televising Counter Terrorism: Torture, Denial, and Exception in the Case of 24', *Continuum: Journal of Media & Cultural Studies*, 25 (2): 213–25.

O'Connor, P. (2020), 'Ita may Well Be Right but All Workers Should Be Thanked', *Canberra Times*, 27 July. Available online: https://www.canberratimes.com.au/story/6849624/ita-may-well-be-right-but-all-workers-should-be-thanked/ (accessed 12 September 2022).

OECD (2021), *OECD Policy Responses to Coronavirus (COVID-19): Supporting Young People's Mental Health through the COVID-19 Crisis*, 12 May. Available online: https://www.oecd.org/coronavirus/policy-responses/supporting-young-people-s-mental-health-through-the-covid-19-crisis-84e143e5/ (accessed 18 September 2022).

OfCom (2020), *Half of UK Adults Exposed to False Claims about Coronavirus*. Available online: https://www.ofcom.org.uk/about-ofcom/latest/featuresand-news/half-of-uk-adults-exposed-to-false-claims-about-coronavirus (accessed 18 July 2022).

Ornstein, C. (2020), 'No, President Trump, the Coronavirus Is Nothing Like H1N1 Swine Flu Either', *ProPublica*, 19 March. Available online: https://www.propublica.org/article/no-president-trump-the-coronavirus-is-nothing-like-h1n1-swine-flu-either (accessed 18 August 2022).

Ortiz, Aimee (2020), 'Man Who Said, "If I Get Corona, I Get Corona," Apologizes', *New York Times*, 24 March. Available online: https://www.nytimes.com/2020/03/24/us/coronavirus-brady-sluder-spring-break.html (accessed 12 September 2022).

Ostherr, K. (2004), ' "Invisible Invaders": The Global Body in Public Health Films', in L. D. Friedman (ed.), *Cultural Sutures: Medicine and Media*, 299–314, Durham, NC: Duke University Press.

Pakman, D. (2021), 'Trump & GOP WRONG, Suicides DOWN in 2020', *YouTube*, 10 April. Available online: https://www.youtube.com/watch?v=56tRmhvgzDs&t=141s&ab_channel=DavidPakmanShow (accessed 11 April 2021).

Palmer, B. (2021), 'Our 1918 Pandemic – The Numbers Then and Now', *Independent*, 27 March. Available online: https://www.marshallindependent.com/opinion/local-columns/2021/03/our-1918-pandemic-the-numbers-then-and-now/#:~:text=Demographers%20estimate%20the%20global%20population,the%20 current%20COVID%2D19%20pandemic (accessed 19 September 2022).

Papacharissi, Z. (2015), *Affective Publics: Sentiment, Technology, and Politics*, Oxford: Oxford University Press.

Paynter, J. (2020), 'Nathan Glover launches Makeshift Security Force for Melbourne Anti-lockdown Protests', *News.com.au*, 17 September. Available online: https://www. news.com.au/technology/online/social/nathan-glover-launches-makeshift-security-force-for-melbourne-antilockdown-protests/news-story/453af5cd551fa347692921c1 b4a38a82 (accessed 17 September 2020).

Penders, B., A. Wolters, E. F. Feskens, F. Brouns, M. Huber, E. Maeckelberghe, G. Navis, T. Ockhuizen, J. Plat, J. Sikkema, M. Stasse-Wolthuis, P. van 't Veer, M. Verweij and J. de Vries (2017), 'Capable and Credible? Challenging Nutrition Science', *European Journal of Nutrition*, 56 (6): 2009–2012.

Petterson, C. (2012), 'Colonial Subjectification: Foucault, Christianity and Governmentality', *Cultural Studies Review*, 18 (2): 89–108.

Piotrowski, Daniel and Brittany Chain (2021). 'How Sydney's Lockdown Broke Dieter Brummer', *Daily Mail Australia*, 1 August. Available online: https://www.dailymail. co.uk/news/article-9841931/Home-Away-Dieter-Brummer-Shane-Parrish-dead-Covid-Sydney-lockdown.html (accessed 1 August 2021).

Plant, B. (2011), 'Welcoming Dogs: Levinas and "the Animal" Question', *Philosophy and Social Criticism*, 27 (1): 49–71.

Poster, M. (2001), 'Citizens, Digital Media and Globalization', *Mots Pluriels*, 18 (1): 1–11.

Poynting, S., G. Noble, P. Tabar and J. Collins (2004), *Bin Laden in the Suburbs: Criminalising the Arab Other*, Sydney, NSW: Sydney Institute of Criminology.

Probyn, E. (2000), *Carnal Appetites: FoodSexIdentities*, London & New York: Routledge.

Probyn, E. (2005), *Blush: Faces of Shame*, Minneapolis, MN: University of Minnesota Press.

Pugliese, J. (2004), 'The Incommensurability of Law to Justice: Refugees and Australia's Temporary Protection Visa', *Law and Literature*, 16 (3): 285–311.

Qasi, M. (2020), 'Building Resilience in COVID-19 Times', *People Matters*, 27 August. Available online: https://www.peoplemattersglobal.com/blog/culture/building-resilience-in-covid-19-times-26789 (accessed 12 September 2022).

Radway, J. (1988), 'Reception Study: Ethnography and the Problems of Dispersed Audiences and Nomadic Subjects', *Cultural Studies*, 2 (4): 359–76.

Raffoul, F. (1998), 'The Subject of the Welcome: On Jacques Derrida's Adieu à Emmanuel Lévinas', *Symposium*, 2 (2): 211–22.

Rancière, J. (2016), 'The Populism That Is Not to Be Found', in A. Badiou, P. Bourdieu, J. Butler, G. Didi-Huberman, S. Khiari and J. Rancière (eds), *What Is a People?* trans. J. Gladding, 101–5, New York: Columbia University Press.

Reicher, S. (2022), 'Boris Johnson's Non-Apology Underlines His Utter Contempt for the British Public', *The Guardian*, 14 January. Available online: https://www.

theguardian.com/commentisfree/2022/jan/13/boris-johnson-british-public-prime-minister-no-10-lockdown-party (accessed 14 January 2022).

Reuters Fact Check (2022), 'Fact Check – Preventing Transmission Never Required for COVID Vaccines' Initial Approval; Pfizer Vax Did Reduce Transmission of Early Variants', *Reuters*, 15 October. Available online: https://www.reuters.com/article/factcheck-pfizer-vaccine-transmission-idUSL1N31F20E (accessed 19 October 2022).

RMIT ABC Fact Check (2021), 'Josh Frydenberg Says Melbourne Is the World's Most Locked Down City. Is That Correct?', *ABC News*, 25 October. Available online: https://www.abc.net.au/news/2021-10-25/fact-check-is-melbourne-most-locked-down-city/100560172 (accessed 12 August 2022).

Romer, D. and K. H. Jamieson (2020), 'Conspiracy Theories as Barriers to Controlling the Spread of COVID-19 in the U.S.', *Social Science & Medicine*, 263 (1): 1–8.

Rosello, M. (1998), *Declining the Stereotype: Ethnicity and Representation in French Cultures*, Hanover, NH: University Press of New England.

Sakkal, P. and S. F. Koob (2022), '"Extremely Disappointed" Novak Djokovic Deported after Losing Visa Battle', *The Age*, 16 January. Available online: https://www.theage.com.au/sport/novak-djokovic-visa-saga-returns-to-federal-court-20220116-p59olc.html (accessed 16 January 2022).

Schehr, R. C. (2005), 'Conventional Risk Discourse and the Proliferation of Fear', *Criminal Justice Policy Review*, 16 (1): 38–58.

Schofield, M. (1976), *Promiscuity*, London: Victor Gollancz Ltd.

Secomb, L. (2007), *Philosophy and Love: From Plato to Popular Culture*, Edinburgh: Edinburgh University Press.

Sedgwick, E. K. (2003), *Touching Feeling: Affect, Pedagogy, Performativity*, Durham, NC: Duke University Press.

Serco Institute (2022), Poll: *Nearly 60% of UK Know Someone Who Broke Lockdown Rules and Majority Sceptical of Sue Gray Investigation Outcomes ahead of Publication*. Available online: https://www.sercoinstitute.com/news/2022/poll-nearly-60-of-the-uk-public-know-someone-who-broke-lockdown-rules-majority-sceptical-of-sue-gray-investigation-outcomes-ahead-of-report-publication (accessed 22 September 2022).

Sharma, S. (2013), 'Critical Time', *Communication and Critical/Cultural Studies*, 10 (2–3): 312–18.

Sharma, S. (2014), 'Because the Night Belongs to Lovers: Occupying the Time of Precarity', *Communication and Critical/Cultural Studies*, 11 (1): 5–14.

Shaw, T. and D. J. Youngblood (2010), *Cinematic Cold War: The American and Soviet Struggle for Hearts and Minds*, Lawrence, KS: University Press of Kansas.

Shelley, M. (1992), *Frankenstein*, London: Penguin Classics.

Shelley, M. (2004), *The Last Man*, London: Wordsworth Editions Ltd.

Shneidman, E. (1985), *Definition of Suicide*, New York: John Wiley & Sons.

Shriver, L. (2003), 'Population in Literature', *Population and Development Review*, 29 (2): 153–62.

Silverstein, A. M. (2009), *A History of Immunology*, second edition. London: Academic Press.

Silverstone, R. (1981), *The Message of Television: Myth and Narrative in Contemporary Culture*, London: Heinemann.

Sims, D. (2020), '22 Movies about the End of the World to Watch Now', *The Atlantic*, 18 April. Available online: https://www.theatlantic.com/culture/archive/2020/04/best-apocalyptic-films-watch-quarantine/610072/ (accessed 19 September 2022).

Singh Grewal, D. (2016), 'Conspiracy Theories in a Networked World', *Critical Review*, 28 (1): 24–43.

Smalley, N., J. Scourfield and K. Greenland (2005), 'Young People, Gender and Suicide: A Review of Research on the Social Context', *Journal of Social Work*, 5 (2): 133–54.

Soneson, E., S. Puntis, N. Chapman, K. L. Mansfield, P. Jones and M. Fazel (2022), 'Happier during Lockdown: A Descriptive Analysis of Self-Reported Wellbeing in 17,000 UK School Students during Covid-19 Lockdown', *European Child & Adolescent Psychiatry*. Available online: https://doi.org/10.17863/CAM.80353 (accessed 12 October 2022).

State of Florida (2020), *Office of the Governor Executive Order Number 20-68 (Emergency Management – COVID-19)*. Available online: https://www.flgov.com/wp-content/uploads/2020/03/EO-20-68.pdf (accessed 12 September 2022).

Tellier, L. (2020), 'Pourquoi le coronavirus n'a pas été créé en laboratoire', *Sciences*, 3 May. Available online: https://www.lefigaro.fr/sciences/pourquoi-le-coronavirus-n-a-pas-ete-cree-en-laboratoire-20200503 (accessed 12 June 2020).

The Care Collective (2020), *The Care Manifesto: The Politics of Interdependence*, London and New York: Verso.

The Economist (2020), 'Only the World Wars Have Rivalled Covid-19 for News Coverage', *The Economist*, 19 December. Available online: https://www.economist.com/graphic-detail/2020/12/19/only-the-world-wars-have-rivalled-covid-19-for-news-coverage (accessed 12 July 2022).

The New Daily (2020), 'Victoria's COVID Toll Rises by 12, Infections Hold Steady', *The New Daily*, 28 August. Available online: https://thenewdaily.com.au/news/coronavirus/2020/08/28/victoria-113-cases-covid/ (accessed 11 April 2021).

Thompson, E. P. (1967), 'Time, Work-Discipline, and Industrial Capitalism', *Past & Present*, 38 (December): 56–97.

Thorpe, V. (2020), 'Balcony Singing in Solidarity Spreads across Italy during Lockdown', *The Guardian*, 15 March. Available online: https://www.theguardian.com/world/2020/mar/14/solidarity-balcony-singing-spreads-across-italy-during-lockdown (accessed 12 May 2021).

Topsfield, J. (2020), 'Kindness Outbreak Keeping People Occupied and Entertained', *The Age*, 16 March. Available online: https://www.theage.com.au/national/victoria/kindness-outbreak-keeping-people-occupied-and-entertained-20200316-p54and.html (accessed 19 March 2020).

Topsfield, J. (2021), 'Generation COVID: Will the Kids Be Alright?', *The Age*, 12 June. Available online: https://www.theage.com.au/national/victoria/generation-covid-will-the-kids-be-alright-20210611-p58048.html (accessed 12 September 2022).

Topsfield, J. and S. Aubrey (2022), 'We're Not "Snowflakes": Why Young People Have It Harder than Ever', *Sydney Morning Herald*, 17 April. Available online: https://www.smh.com.au/lifestyle/health-and-wellness/we-re-not-snowflakes-why-young-people-have-it-harder-than-ever-20220413-p5ad61.html (accessed 10 September 2022).

Topsfield, J. and R. Millar (2021), 'How Denise Morgan Escaped Albert Park's House of Horrors', *The Age*, 27 September. Available online: https://www.theage.com.au/national/victoria/how-denise-morgan-escaped-melbourne-s-house-of-horrors-20210920-p58t25.html (accessed 27 September 2021).

Tronto, J. C. (2013), *Caring Democracy: Markets, Equality, and Justice*, New York: New York University Press.

Tuohy, W. (2020), 'It Feels Surreal in the Suburbs Now I Cannot See Your Face', *The Age*, 26 July. Available online: https://www.theage.com.au/national/victoria/it-feels-surreal-in-the-suburbs-now-i-cannot-see-your-face-20200724-p55f5i.html (accessed 27 July 2020).

Tuohy, W. (2021), 'Disruption to "Sense of Self" Contributed to Pandemic-Linked Suicides', *The Age*, 14 August. Available online: https://www.theage.com.au/national/victoria/disruption-to-sense-of-self-contributed-to-pandemic-linked-suicides-20210813-p58ie4.html (accessed 14 August 2021).

Turner, G. (1993), 'Media Texts and Messages', in S. Cunningham and G. Turner (eds), *The Media in Australia: Industries, Texts, Audiences*, 205–66, St. Leonards, NSW: Allen & Unwin.

Turner, L. and A. Evans (2020), 'Coronavirus: How to Grieve a Loved One When You Can't Say Goodbye', *BBC News*, 4 April. Available online: https://www.bbc.com/news/uk-52142660 (accessed 9 October 2022).

Turner, V. (1969), *The Ritual Process: Structure and Anti-structure*, Chicago: Aldine.

Turton-Turner, P. (2007), 'The Role of Ridicule in Naked Charity Calendars', *Continuum: Journal of Media & Cultural Studies*, 21 (3): 419–32.

UK Department of Health and Social Care (2020), *Guidance: Making a Support Bubble with Another Household*. Available online: https://www.gov.uk/guidance/making-a-support-bubble-with-another-household (accessed 12 October 2022).

Unger, M. (2012a), 'Introduction to the Volume', in M. Unger (ed.), *The Social Ecology of Resilience: A Handbook of Theory and Practice*, 1–9, New York: Springer.

Unger, M. (2012b), 'Social Ecologies and Their Contribution to Resilience', in M. Unger (ed.), *The Social Ecology of Resilience: A Handbook of Theory and Practice*, 13–31, New York: Springer.

Uniting NSW (2020), *Six Ways to Care for Your Mental Health during COVID-19*. Available online: https://www.uniting.org/blog-newsroom/uniting-life/wellbeing/six-ways-to-care-for-your-mental-health-during-covid-19- (accessed 12 July 2022).

Urry, J. (2007), *Mobilities*, Cambridge: Polity.

Victor, D., L. Serviss and A. Paybarah (2020), 'In His Own Words, Trump on the Coronavirus and Masks', *New York Times*, 2 October. Available online: https://www.nytimes.com/2020/10/02/us/politics/donald-trump-masks.html (accessed 9 July 2022).

Vigni, L. (2001), 'Smallpox Vaccination in Siena during the Napoleonic Era', *Le Infezioni in Medicina*, 9 (2): 115.

Watson, O. J., G. Barnsley, J. Toor, A. B. Hogan, P. Winskill and A. C. Ghani (2022), 'Global Impact of the First Year of COVID-19 Vaccination: A Mathematical Modelling Study', *The Lancet Infectious Diseases*, 22 (9): 1293–302.

Wenger, E. (1998), *Communities of Practice: Learning, Meaning, and Identity*, Cambridge: Cambridge University Press.

Wexler, L. M., G. DiFluvio and T. K. Burke (2009), 'Resilience and Marginalized Youth: Making a Case for Personal and Collective Meaning-Making as Part of Resilience Research in Public Health', *Social Science & Medicine*, 69 (2009): 565–70.

Wheaton, B. (2000), ' "New Lads"?: Masculinities and the "New Sport" Participant', *Men and Masculinities*, 2 (4): 434–56.

White, J., I. Marsh, M. J. Kral and J. Morris (2016), 'Rethinking Suicide', in J. White, I. Marsh, M. J. Kral and J. Morris (eds), *Critical Suicidology: Transforming Suicide Research and Prevention for the 21st Century*, 1–11, Vancouver: University of British Columbia Press.

Wiegman, R. and E. A. Wilson (2015), 'Introduction: Antinormativity's Queer Conventions', *Differences: A Journal of Feminist Cultural Studies*, 26 (1): 1–25.

Williams, R. (1990), 'The Technology and the Society', in D. Bennett (ed.), *Popular Fiction: Technology, Ideology, Production, Reading*, 9–22, London: Routledge.

Woodward, K. (2002), *Understanding Identity*, London: Arnold.

World Health Organization (2020a), *WHO Director-General's Opening Remarks at the Media Briefing on COVID-19 – 11 March 2020*. Available online: https://www.who.int/director-general/speeches/detail/who-director-general-s-opening-remarks-at-the-media-briefing-on-covid-19---11-march-2020 (accessed 12 August 2022).

World Health Organization (2020b), *Novel Coronavirus (2019-nCoV) Situation Report, 13*. Available online: https://www.who.int/docs/default-source/coronaviruse/situation-reports/20200202-sitrep-13-ncov-v3.pdf (accessed 18 September 2022).

World Health Organization (2022), *COVID-19: Physical Distancing.* Available online: https://www.who.int/westernpacific/emergencies/covid-19/information/physical-distancing (accessed 30 September 2022).

Wren, J. (2020), 'Wren's Week: Victoria Overcomes with Premier Andrews" Leadership"', *Independent Australia*, 31 October. Available online: https://independentaustralia. net/politics/politics-display/wrens-week-victoria-overcomes-with-premier-andrews-leadership,14466 (accessed 31 October 2020).

Wyn, J. and D. Woodman (2006), 'Generation, Youth and Social Change in Australia', *Journal of Youth Studies*, 9 (5): 495–514.

Index

www.ingramcontent.com/pod-product-compliance
Lightning Source LLC
Chambersburg PA
CBHW050712280326
41926CB00088B/3001